TRANSFORM

MAYO CLINIC PLATFORM AND THE DIGITAL FUTURE OF HEALTH

TRANSFORM

PAUL CERRATO, MA • JOHN D. HALAMKA, MD, MS

MAYO CLINIC | Press

Proceeds from the sale of every book benefit important medical research and education at Mayo Clinic.

To stay informed about Mayo Clinic Press, please subscribe to our free e-newsletter at MCPress.MayoClinic.org or follow us on social media. For bulk sales, contact Mayo Clinic at SpecialSalesMayoBooks@mayo.edu.

Image Credits All photographs and illustrations are copyright of Mayo Foundation for Medical Education and Research (MFMER) except for the following: p. 105 / National Human Genome Research Institute / genome.gov

MAYO CLINIC PRESS
200 First St. SW
Rochester, MN 55905
MCPress.MayoClinic.org

ISBN: 979-8-88770-326-8 (paperback)
      979-8-88770-327-5 (ebook)

Library of Congress Control Number: 2024060107

Library of Congress Cataloging-in-Publication Data is available upon request.

Printed in the United States

First printing: 2025

There is honor love and family
And work left to be done.

—Livingston Taylor

Contents

Introduction

People pick up books about digital health for a variety of reasons. Some do it because they're looking to technology to identify better treatment for a medical condition. Others want to use the latest digital tools to stay healthy, or conversely, because they have perplexing signs and symptoms for which they're seeking a definitive diagnosis. And still others have heard about the possible benefits of artificial intelligence (AI) or read about new software programs purported to detect disorders that are usually missed during a conventional medical workup.

Whatever your reason for delving into this book, our goal is to provide you with an optimistic yet realistic picture of what digital health can do for individuals and for the population as a whole. Several of the patient stories in the chapters to come will give you a sense of just how powerful digital tools are. You'll learn about:

- Peter Maercklein, a retired financial executive whose irregular, fluttering heartbeat was diagnosed with the help of an AI-powered algorithm;

- Ken Counihan, whose blood clots were diagnosed with the help of his Apple Watch;

- Trixie Scott, a woman whose brain disorder was diagnosed with the help of AI-driven technology; and

- Amy Satterfield, a yoga instructor whose smartwatch helped uncover the valve problem that caused her heart to fail.

Of course, like all new technology, digital health tools also can be misused, and their value can be exaggerated by entrepreneurs who don't have scientific evidence to back up their claims. For example, some people say that AI-based programs can replace physicians or advanced practice providers by making more accurate diagnoses and treatment recommendations. Those claims are exaggerated. So, too, are some claims that have been made about what telemedicine consultations can accomplish, which prompted the U.S. Department of Justice to coordinate law enforcement efforts to rein in fraud in this area.[1]

To take full advantage of the latest healthcare technology and help doctors and patients separate the wheat from the chaff, Mayo Clinic created the Mayo Clinic Platform (MCP). It enables Mayo Clinic to expand beyond our walls, multiply what we can do on our own, and innovate in new ways to touch the lives of millions of people. Through a coordinated portfolio of initiatives, MCP is unlocking the ever-increasing potential of technology and Big Data to make connections and innovate in new ways.

These initiatives are having a global impact through wearables, machine learning, and AI. In conjunction with best-in-class partners from across the world, MCP is launching a portfolio of high-impact, transformative platform ventures that will make Mayo's expertise available globally. These efforts will harness Big Data and AI to create insights that are both personalized and powered by millions of data points. MCP combines cutting-edge data science, analytics, innovation, and business applications. This engine, fortified with patient-centric security and privacy mechanisms, is designed to uncover cures, enable precise and personalized treatments, and transform care.

With this transformation in mind, Mayo Clinic has joined with more than 1,000 other healthcare organizations to ensure that AI is used responsibly. Called the Coalition for Health AI (CHAI), it's a community of academic health systems, organizations, and expert AI and data science practitioners. These members have come together to harmonize standards and reporting for health AI and to educate end users on how to evaluate these technologies to drive their adoption.

THE ROAD AHEAD

In Chapters 1 and 2, we'll explain how digital health tools, such as a massive data bank of patient information derived from electronic health records and other sources, are being developed. This treasure trove of de-identified patient data is being used to develop algorithms to improve diagnosis and treatment—with patient permission, of course.

Chapter 3 describes the guardrails being created to make sure that all the data and algorithms are safe and effective. In Chapter 4, we'll explain the specific digital solutions being developed. Figure 1 is a snapshot of what these solutions look like. They include software systems that improve detection of colorectal cancer and cardiovascular problems and a "hospital at home" program that goes far beyond the visiting nurse services that most people think of when they hear about home care.

In Chapter 5, we'll talk about the epidemic of misdiagnosis that is affecting millions of people around the globe—as well as solutions to address the problem. A report from the National Academy of Medicine (NAM) points out that every year, about 5% of adult outpatients in the United States experience a diagnostic error.[2] According to the NAM report, diagnostic mishaps contribute to about 1 in 10 patient deaths, cause as much as 17% of adverse effects seen in hospitalized patients, and affect approximately 12 million adult outpatients a year, which translates into 1 in 20 Americans. About 71,400 of the 850,000 patients who die in U.S. hospitals every year had a significant health condition that went undetected.

Chapter 6 covers one of the most exciting developments in medicine: the new role that genomics is beginning to play in treating genetic disorders that were once thought to be uncurable, such as sickle cell anemia, muscular dystrophy, and cystic fibrosis.

In Chapter 7, we explore the profound impact that social factors have on a person's health. As the Centers for Disease Control and Prevention points out: "Health is influenced by many factors, which may generally be organized into five broad categories known as determinants of health: genetics, behavior, environmental and physical influences, medical care and social factors. These five categories are interconnected."[3] So-called social determinants of health have been overlooked by most healthcare providers over the decades. They encompass economic and social conditions that influence the health of people and communities. These conditions are shaped by socioeconomic position, which is the amount of money, power, and resources

FIGURE 1

AI-driven solutions at Mayo Clinic Platform to improve and transform care

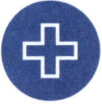

Advanced Care at Home

In partnership with Medically Home, a model for delivering complex care to patients from the comfort of home has transformed the future of medical care delivery.

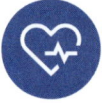

Cardiology AI

In collaboration with partner Anumana, several AI-enabled algorithms that detect heart diseases earlier.

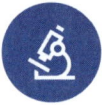

Early Disease Detection

Using AI-driven technology, these solutions will help identify patients at risk for colorectal cancer, diabetes and opioid use disorder.

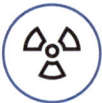

Radiology AI

An AI algorithm to auto-contour head and neck cancers that has been proven superior and more efficient to current software tools and clinical approaches.

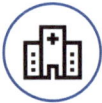

Gastroenterology & Hepatology AI

A digital endoscopy platform that automates image and video acquisition, integrates the data into EHRs so clinicians can access an endoscopy video library.

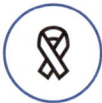

Oncology Care

Using deep learning techniques, test results, genetics, and benign breast biopsy findings are harnessed to better identify women at high risk for breast cancer.

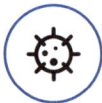

Digital Pathology

Digitized and stored pathology slides from patients to fuel better access for providers, educators, and researchers.

that people have, all of which are influenced by socioeconomic and political factors (e.g., policies, culture, and societal values). An individual's socioeconomic position can be shaped by various factors, such as their education, occupation, or income. All these factors (social determinants) impact the health and well-being of people and the communities they interact with.

Finally, in Chapter 8, we'll dive into the most talked-about branch of digital health: chatbots and generative AI. These new tools have captured the public's attention with their ability to carry on long humanlike conversations, create novel images, and write poetry and computer code. In healthcare, they are being explored for their potential to streamline routine administrative tasks, answer patient emails, and perhaps even improve physicians' ability to make more informed diagnoses. But as the chapter will demonstrate, chatbots also can wreak havoc, misleading patients and healthcare professionals with fabricated data.

It is not an exaggeration to say that we're entering a new era in medicine, one in which digital health will profoundly impact the ways you and your neighbors receive patient care and provide medical self-care. While it may be true that medical professionals will not be replaced by the technologies we talk about in this book, professionals who embrace these innovations will replace those who do not.

A NOTE TO OUR READERS

Our hope for this book is to reach patients and consumers who want to better understand digital health; however, there is also much information that will interest healthcare professionals and technologists. With that in mind, we have also included several sections labeled TechStop, which provide a deeper dive into many of the topics in the book.

At the time of writing, all sources cited in this book were publicly available. However, the availability of online health information can change over time, so if a link is no longer accessible, consider checking the organization's main website or searching for updated resources.

References

|1| U.S. Department of Justice. Justice Department Charges Dozens for $1.2 Billion in Health Care Fraud; July 20, 2022. Accessed October 23, 2023. https://www .justice.gov/opa/pr/justice-department-charges-dozens-12-billion-health-care -fraud.

|2| Committee on Diagnostic Error in Health Care; Board on Health Care Services; Institute of Medicine; The National Academies of Sciences, Engineering, and Medicine. Balogh EP, Miller BT, Ball JR, eds. *Improving Diagnosis in Health Care*. National Academies Press (US); December 29, 2015. Accessed November 6, 2023. https://pubmed.ncbi.nlm.nih.gov/26803862/.

|3| Centers for Disease Control and Prevention. Social Determinants of Health; December 19, 2019. Accessed November 7, 2023. https://www.cdc.gov/health -disparities-hiv-std-tb-hepatitis/about/social-determinants-of-health.html.

CHAPTER 1

Building the network

In our Introduction, we briefly mentioned Peter Maercklein, a retired financial executive in his early seventies who discovered he had atrial fibrillation (AFib)—irregular fluttering heartbeats that can lead to blood clots—with the help of an artificial intelligence (AI)-powered algorithm. Like many people with AFib, Peter didn't feel symptoms. He and his wife were enjoying retirement in southeastern Minnesota, traveling often in their RV and spending much of the summer up north in Grand Marais. In 2020, Mayo Clinic coordinators in Rochester asked him to participate in a research study. Now complete and published,[1] that study evaluated AI-guided screening for AFib using electrocardiograms (ECGs) taken during normal heart rhythm to identify previously unrecognized AFib. Peter's AI-ECG showed he had an 81.49% probability of experiencing AFib, so he was outfitted with a Holter monitor to record his heart rhythm over time. Within a few days, the monitor confirmed that Peter had AFib while he was walking on a treadmill at home. He saw his care team and had further testing to confirm the diagnosis, and then went on a blood thinner medication to reduce his risk of having a stroke. Later, Peter had a pacemaker implanted to control his heart rhythm.

Dr. Paul Friedman, one of the cardiologists involved in the study evaluating the benefits of using AI to detect AFib, points out that cardiovascular disease is the number 1 killer in the United States and worldwide, and that many cases of AFib are preventable. What if we could detect problems earlier and head off disease instead of waiting for a life-altering event like a heart attack, cardiac arrest, or stroke? That's exactly what's happening at Mayo Clinic and other leading medical centers around the world. Mayo Clinic uses AI to detect and predict heart disease using ECG readings, which are common, relatively inexpensive, and can also be obtained from wearable technology such as a smartwatch. AI can discern electrocardiographic changes that the human eye can't, picking up electrical signatures of heart disease even before symptoms appear.

Mayo Clinic created an AI-ECG dashboard viewable in the electronic health record (EHR) that shows a patient's probability of certain heart conditions such as AFib, low ejection fraction (weak heart pump), hypertrophic cardiomyopathy, or HCM (a thickening of the left ventricle, the lower main pumping chamber of the heart), aortic stenosis (calcification in the arteries), and amyloidosis, which involves a buildup of folded proteins. The dashboard provides multiple points for diagnosis, prognosis, and clinical care orchestration. Clinicians can compare AI evaluations of a patient's ECGs over time and quickly get a wide-lens view of the person's heart and circulatory system health. Patients can even send Apple Watch ECGs directly to their EHRs via a secure Mayo Clinic app, adding another checkpoint for monitoring changes. This information adds to a clinician's knowledge and can be used to flag patients who need further testing and, potentially, therapy.

The advantage of AI is more far-reaching than many people realize. It is making innovative medical care more democratic. Across the United States and globally, not everyone has access to a large medical center with specialized diagnostics. The symptoms of some heart diseases are common to other conditions, so how do we more quickly and easily identify patients who need care? AI-ECG algorithms offer a relatively inexpensive way to spot disease and profile individuals who are at increased risk for heart disease. These investigational tools are being used as a guide at Mayo Clinic, and they're being reviewed by regulators for broader commercial use. Once approved, we anticipate that these algorithms will be widely available and adopted globally to improve diagnosis and patient health.

While the value of AI-fueled algorithms is obvious, what often goes unnoticed is the collection of patient information—a massive dataset—that enables researchers to develop these digital tools in the first place. Without this data bank, it would be nearly impossible to conduct the clinical trials used to create the algorithms.

THE POWER OF LARGE NUMBERS

The data network that Mayo Clinic uses contains tens of millions of electronic patient records that can be tapped to gain insights into what causes specific diseases and how best to treat them. This is all part of the Big Data movement that has gained momentum in medicine in recent years. The value of such large numbers is amply illustrated by investigations into possible harms caused by certain prescription drugs. Typically, such medications are tested among a few thousand subjects in clinical trials. Unfortunately, patient populations of this size are often not large enough to detect relatively uncommon adverse effects.

A good example of the power of large numbers is a study conducted by David J. Graham, MD, MPH, the U.S. Food and Drug Administration (FDA) Associate Director for Science, Office of Drug Safety, and his associates. They analyzed records from approximately 1.4 million patients who were members of Kaiser Permanente in California. The aim of the research was to determine if rofecoxib (Vioxx), a cyclooxygenase 2 (COX-2) selective nonsteroidal anti-inflammatory drug, increased the risk of acute myocardial infarction—a type of heart attack—and sudden cardiac death. Graham and associates were able to review the equivalent of 2,302,029 person-years of follow-up. In this population, they detected 8,142 cases of serious coronary heart disease (CHD), 2,210 of which were fatal. The patients taking any dose of the medication were 59% more likely to develop CHD than the controls.[2] In patients who took 25 mg/day or less, the odds of developing CHD were 47% higher. Finally, among patients who took high doses, namely more than 25 mg daily, the odds of heart disease were 258% higher.

Several smaller, earlier studies published before the FDA data were available suggested an association between Vioxx and heart disease, but those findings had several shortcomings. The data from Graham and associates, which were presented at a conference before being published in *The Lancet,* made headlines and embroiled the researchers in a confrontation with FDA officials, who initially didn't want the results made public.[3] Vioxx was withdrawn from the market by Merck on September 30, 2004. But estimates indicate that, during the time the drug was on the market, more than 100 million prescriptions were written and between 88,000 and 140,000 excess cases of serious CHD may have resulted from the public's exposure to Vioxx. Its removal was clearly a testament to the value of Big Data. The Graham study is only one of many that illustrate the benefits of using massive datasets to glean meaningful insights about healthcare.[4]

Large data networks have captured the attention of healthcare executives and clinicians. They're part of the Big Data movement and a related specialty, data analytics. Big Data is usually distinguished from "small data" by its volume, velocity, and variety. The so-called 3-Vs reflect the fact that the amount of data available for analysis is huge, compared with the quantity of data that has traditionally been obtained from clinical trials and population studies. The databases currently being examined may include petabytes of data, which each contain 1,024 terabytes, or exabytes, which each contain 1,024 petabytes. (A terabyte contains 1,024 gigabytes.) They may comprise billions of patient records, such as EHR data, social media, claims data, and much more. The databases typically consist of structured data—for example, the ICD (International Classification of Diseases) codes for patients—and unstructured data such as narratives describing patients' signs and symptoms. The speed or velocity with which these data are accumulating and at which they can be moved from place to place also distinguishes Big Data from more traditional sources of patient information, as does the variety of types of data, which can include input from remote sensors, text data on hard drives and smartphones, and imaging data from videos, photographs, and X-rays, among others.[4]

All the data can be saved in different types of "storage bins," including relational databases and data warehouses, and analyzed by linking the bins through a process called distributed computing, using a tool such as Hadoop (pronounced huh-DOOP). Data scientists also use terms such as "semantics," "syntax," and "ontology," all of which have special meanings in the context of medical informatics.

In a simple computer file folder or directory, you might store information in individual files as Microsoft Office text documents or PDFs, and images as TIFF or JPEG files. But if you tried to identify relationships, correlations, or patterns between these diverse collections of data, it would be difficult. Relational databases help solve this problem, making analysis easier by creating a schema, which is the structural representation of data in a database. The data are compartmentalized in various tables, fields, rows, and columns, and the database creates relationships among the numerous data points. The database then can be queried to pull out links between elements such as columns and rows. One table may list all of a patient's demographic details, including age, address, gender, and race, and a second may list their family medical history. By querying the database, you might be able to determine, for example, which female patients have a history of a specific disease because linkages between the demographics and family history tables are built into the tool.

Understanding the concept of distributed computing is another piece of the puzzle that can make Big Data less mysterious. In the simplest terms, distributed computing is a way for individual computers to talk to one another and function as one gigantic "brain" despite the fact that the machines may be located all over the world. The internet is a distributed computing network, connected by nodes, routers, and the like. Hadoop is another. It's currently being used by data analysts to gain insights from amounts of data that are too massive to be stored economically in any one location.

KATHY HALAMKA'S JOURNEY

All this talk about relational databases, distributed computing, and querying databases may sound esoteric and irrelevant to patients and consumers who are trying to understand how digital health is going to improve their everyday lives. The experiences of Kathy Halamka (John's wife)[4] make the connection obvious. In 2011, Kathy was diagnosed with stage 3 breast cancer, and a sentinel node biopsy revealed that her tumor had already spread to a few nearby lymph nodes. The malignancy was estrogen- and progesterone-positive but HER2-negative, less than 5 cm in diameter, poorly differentiated, and fast growing. According to the American Cancer Society, on average, the 5-year relative survival rate for women like Kathy is 72%, which means that people who have the cancer are only about 72% as likely as people who do not have it to live for at least 5 years after being diagnosed. The standard of care for cases like this is typically chemotherapy followed by mastectomy. But having access to a Big Data database gave her and her oncology team new options and an opportunity to test-drive the personalized medicine approach to healthcare. The database they used was an open-source software platform that gives clinicians and researchers Web-based access to a hospital's EHR, a resource that has the potential to identify treatment options not yet available in the current medical literature or mentioned in official practice guidelines.

Typically, patients like Kathy are treated with a combination of doxorubicin (Adriamycin), cyclophosphamide (Cytoxan), and paclitaxel (Taxol). But a search of the database revealed that many of them developed neuropathy—numbness of the hands and feet—from Taxol. Further investigation found that there was only one clinical trial looking at treatment with Taxol for Kathy's type of cancer, and it used a specific number of milligrams per

kilogram of body weight administered in 9 doses. There were no data to indicate whether this was the optimal dosage regimen or if 3 doses or 11 doses
would have resulted in better outcomes in terms of tumor shrinkage or
adverse effects.

With these findings in hand, Kathy's oncology team decided to personalize
her treatment by administering full protocols of Adriamycin and Cytoxan
but only a half protocol of Taxol, giving her 5 doses rather than 9. This individualized approach caused her tumor to melt away and resulted in minimal
numbness in her hands and feet—an important benefit, considering that
she's a visual artist who relies on her fine motor skills.

MAYO CLINIC'S APPLICATION OF BIG DATA

Mayo Clinic has taken advantage of this Big Data approach to healthcare
by developing a service called Mayo Clinic Platform_Connect. It's a distributed data network through which Mayo partners with health systems,
payers, medical device companies, and academic medical centers to enable
better diagnosis, treatment, and even prevention of disease. Through Mayo
Clinic Platform_Connect, clinical data are connected in a *federated, secure
architecture* to drive innovation in healthcare. (For more details about
what these terms mean, see "How to protect sensitive patient data" on
page 22.)

Every partner in Mayo Clinic Platform_Connect is committed to transforming care with a network of connected data. Each of them brings
unmatched depth and breadth of clean, curated, de-identified data related
to complex and rare health conditions; a wide range of treatments and
therapies; and representation from diverse communities in urban and
rural settings. As this book went to press, five healthcare organizations
were contributing to the Mayo Clinic Platform_Connect dataset, as illustrated in Figure 1.1.

With a globally connected data network, the possibilities are endless. Mayo
Clinic Platform_Connect links de-identified clinical data that will help create
a more efficient system for diagnosis and treatment. It enables clinicians to
deliver better patient care by learning from data from past patients to guide
the care journeys of future patients. Data from geographically and ethnically
diverse patient populations will help create more tailored medicine, healthcare products, services, and solutions. That's not all—large amounts of data
will give scientists a wealth of information for research, including about
rare, serious, and complex diseases.

FIGURE 1.1

The first comprehensive healthcare platform

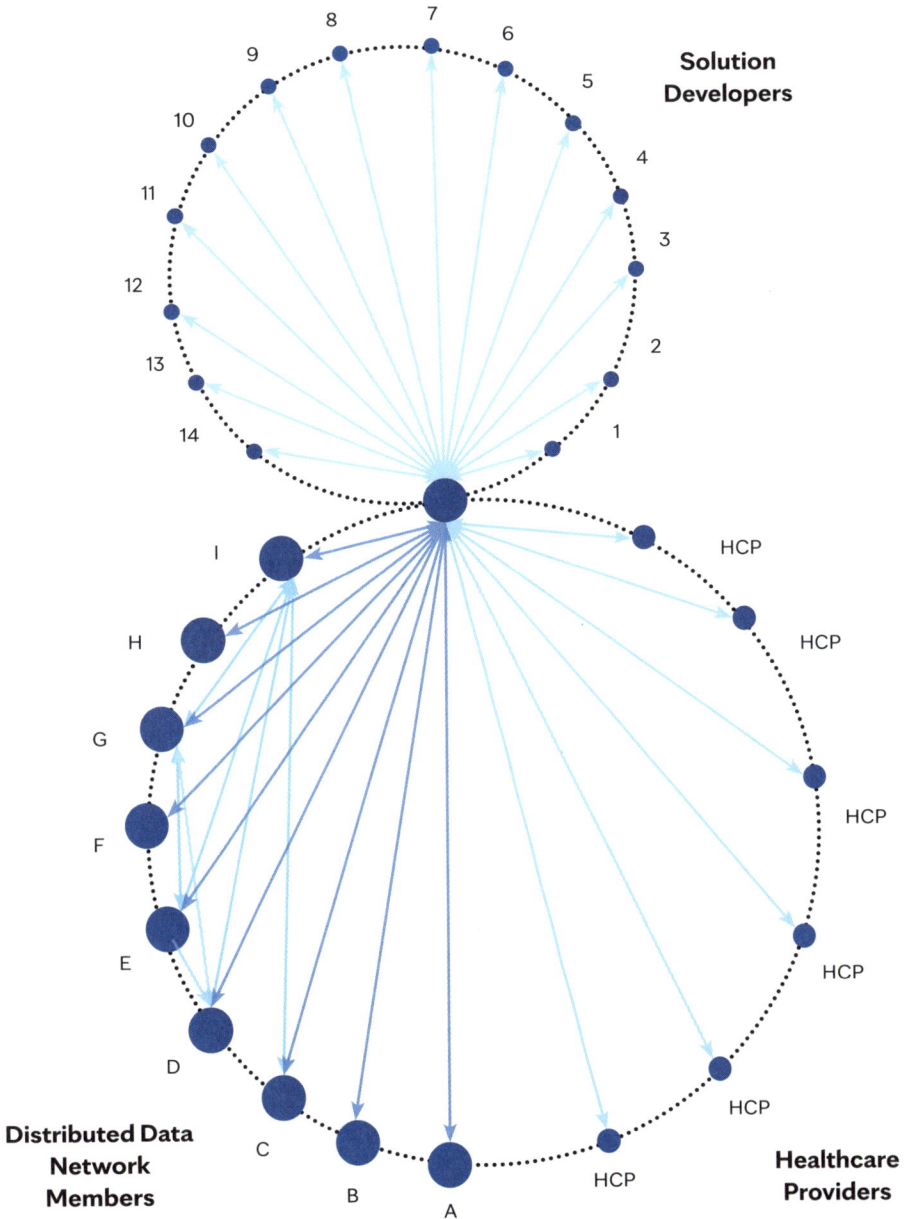

This graphic illustrates the many solution developers that have created algorithms and related services for healthcare providers (HCPs). These solutions are distributed to the HCPs that are part of Mayo Clinic Platform_Connect.

Managing patient data requires a system that enables users to gain insights while at the same time keeping the information private and secure. Mayo Clinic uses a federated approach for this purpose. According to Nvidia, which specializes in high-end computer chips, "Federated learning is a way to develop and validate AI models from diverse data sources while mitigating the risk of compromising data security or privacy, as the data never leaves individual sites."[5] With the federated approach, each source sends their updated model's weights or parameters to a shared virtual location and then the central server aggregates them. That's the approach that Mayo Clinic Platform uses for the Mayo Clinic Platform_Connect dataset.

Given the increasing complexity of healthcare data and the resulting questions surrounding what constitutes adequate de-identification (such as for genetic or radiographic data),* the reality of accessing data has only become more challenging. The optimal solution would incorporate:

- Automated, real-time de-identification such that the most recent data are de-identified without the need for human engagement;

- Technology-based governance to mitigate the risk of re-identifying individuals;

- The ability to operationalize the data so they can be used to train diagnostic and prediction models accurately with minimal computer workload or additional hardware; and

- The ability to scale the approach across any amount of data, regardless of where the data are located and whether they are structured or unstructured.

Creating the model depends on access to clinical data (available in unstructured form, extracted from the EHR), imaging data (computed tomography

---

* De-identification refers to the process of removing and changing the data so that any identifying content is obscured, preventing viewers from linking the content to a specific patient, for instance. U.S. Health Insurance Portability and Accountability Act (HIPAA) regulations include 18 identifiers that must be removed from a patient record to prevent viewers from recognizing who is being discussed. Those identifiers include name, Social Security number, addresses, and a variety of other markers. Mayo Clinic goes even further in its de-identification process to keep patient data private.

scans of the lungs, for example), and genomic data, which together would involve several hundred gigabytes to terabytes.

Mayo Clinic is using a federated model that includes a multilayered defense referred to as Data Behind Glass. The concept of Data Behind Glass is that the de-identified data are stored in an encrypted container, always under control of Mayo Clinic Cloud. Authorized cloud subtenants can be granted access so that their tools can access the de-identified data for algorithm development, but no data can be taken out of the container. This prevents merging the data with other, external data sources.

We've developed a de-identification approach that takes patient privacy to the next level, using a protocol for EHR clinical notes that includes attention-based deep learning models, rule-based methods, and heuristics. Karthik Murugadoss and associates explain that "rule-based systems use pattern matching rules, regular expressions, and dictionary and public database look-ups to identify PII [personally identifiable information] elements."[6] The problem with relying solely on such rules is that they miss things, especially in narrative notes in an EHR, which often include nonstandard expressions, such as unusual spellings and typographical errors. The rules also take a great deal of time to manually create. Traditional machine learning-based systems, too, have their shortcomings.

The ensemble approach used at Mayo includes a next-generation algorithm that incorporates natural language processing and machine learning (see page 25.) When protected health information is detected, the system transforms the identifiers into plausible, though fictional, surrogates to further hide any leaked identifier. We evaluated the system with a publicly available dataset of 515 notes from the de-identification challenge and a dataset of 10,000 notes from Mayo Clinic. We compared our approach with other existing tools considered best-in-class. The results indicated a recall of 0.992 and 0.994 and a precision of 0.979 and 0.967 on the i2b2 and the Mayo Clinic data, respectively.

While this protocol has many advantages over older systems, it's only one component of a more comprehensive system used at Mayo to keep patient data private and secure.

Of course, publicity about data banks naturally leads many people to worry about whether the tools will compromise their personal health information or result in it being shared without their approval. Patient privacy is a top concern for Mayo Clinic. In fact, Mayo Clinic Platform_Connect leads the charge in data privacy and security. Mayo Clinic neither owns nor wants to own the data from our partners. As a result, de-identified clinical data from each partner in Mayo Clinic Platform_Connect stay in that partner's local environment, ensuring that the data remain safe and secure.

All Mayo Clinic Platform_Connect partners operate within Mayo Clinic Platform's Data Behind Glass model. Data Behind Glass is a proprietary system of technical and administrative controls to ensure that privacy and confidentiality are respected and preserved across the distributed data network.

PRIMER ON ALGORITHMS, LANGUAGE PROCESSING AND MACHINE LEARNING

Data scientists and other computer specialists routinely use the terms "algorithm," "language processing," and "machine learning" when discussing many of the new digital tools designed to improve patient health and facilitate diagnosis and treatment of many diseases. You will encounter these terms throughout the book. To appreciate the value of these digital tools, it's worth spending a few minutes to understand what they mean.

Algorithm

A global leader in digital skills development training courses describes an algorithm this way: "An algorithm is a set of commands that must be followed for a computer to perform calculations or other problem-solving operations. According to its formal definition, an algorithm is a finite set of instructions carried out in a specific order to perform a particular task."[7] More basically, an algorithm is a flowchart or roadmap that includes several forks in the road that invite you to go one way or the other, depending on the situation at hand. Businesses and healthcare organizations have used them for decades to make important decisions, even before computers were in the picture.

In medicine, an algorithm or flowchart might start with a woman who has lower right-side abdominal pain. At the first fork in the road, the clinician would be asked: Does the patient have stable vital signs or not? If the answer is stable, the next prompt would be to do a series of lab tests or imaging studies. More pivot points would follow, eventually leading to a final diagnosis. In the case of the woman with lower right-side abdominal pain, the diagnosis might be acute appendicitis, but it could also be a gynecologic disorder, depending on how the questions in the flowchart are answered.

In digital health, an algorithm has a similar function, but it's more likely to be a set of rules for how to detect a spam email to prevent hackers from breaking into a hospital's computer network, for example, or a set of instructions to enable a smartwatch to detect an abnormal heart rhythm, or make it easy for a patient to communicate their blood glucose readings to their advanced practice provider.

Until recently, most algorithms were rule-based, which required programmers to type in lines of computer code that instructed the device to take certain actions. For example, Deep Blue, the IBM computer that defeated Garry Kasparov, then the world chess champion, in 1997, was programmed with millions of moves. Such "old-school" algorithms have been replaced with machine learning systems that seem to "think for themselves."

Machine learning

This is a type of AI. More specifically, machine learning is an AI application that enables the computer program to automatically learn and improve from experience without being explicitly programmed. A good example is a program developed by Google DeepMind called AlphaGo. It, too, is capable of beating chess champions, but it accomplishes that feat by playing thousands of games and learning from them to develop a winning strategy, as opposed to being programmed with previous chess moves.

With deep learning, which is a subset of machine learning, artificial neural networks do the self-learning. As we've pointed out in our earlier books, a neural network that assists in the detection of diabetic retinopathy, a complication that causes blindness, is one of the best examples of this type of machine learning. Similarly, there are networks capable of distinguishing between melanomas and ordinary moles.

Figure 1.2 shows how neural networks are being used to detect skin cancer.[8] They scan tens of thousands of images to learn how to recognize small differences between normal and abnormal skin growths. The "neurons" are nodes or layers that are connected to one another, and as each node is excited by data coming from a digital image, those data are sent to the next

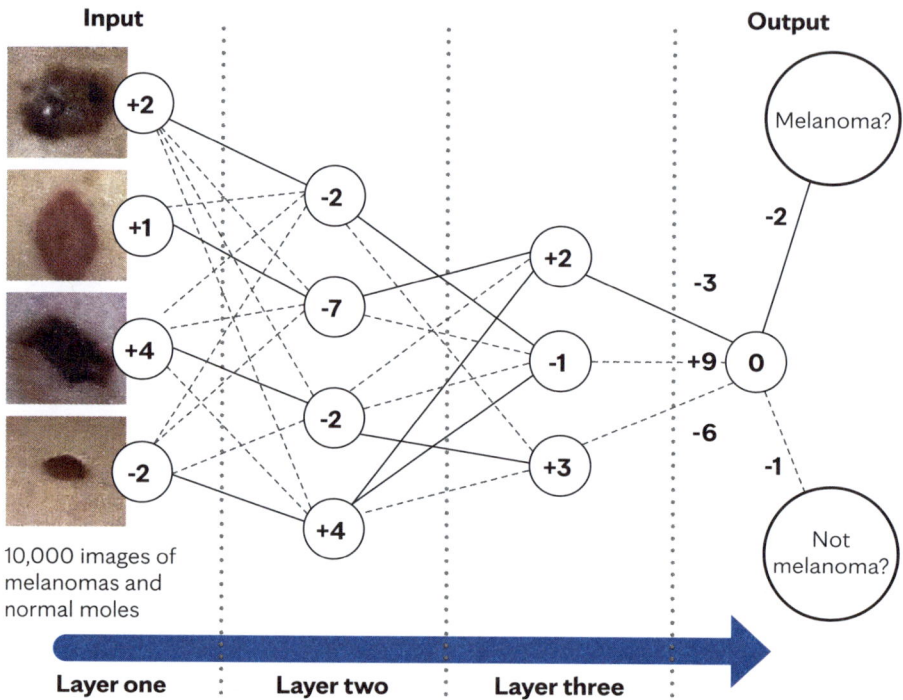

FIGURE 1.2
How neural networks work

Source: Cerrato P, Halamka J. *Redefining the Boundaries of Medicine.*
Mayo Clinic Press; 2023.8

node. The excitement transferred from one node to the next is represented by a specific number or weight. In the case of the skin cancer algorithm, the excitement is the result of the network analyzing millions of pixels in each image. Data representing the pixels in an image are sent through nodes in the first input layer and then transferred to the next layer. The strength of each signal is indicated by a specific numerical value. The goal is to arrive at an output—in this case, a conclusion that the image represents either a melanoma or a normal mole.

Natural language processing

Computers are designed to read a binary language that consists of long strings of 0s and 1s. Because humans don't speak that language, we need a way to bridge the gap, which is where natural language processing (NLP) comes in. IBM explains that NLP is "the branch of computer science—and more specifically, the branch of AI—concerned with giving computers the ability to understand text and spoken words in much the same way human beings can. NLP combines computational linguistics—rule-based modeling of human language—with statistical, machine learning, and deep learning models. Together, these technologies enable computers to process human language in the form of text or voice data and to 'understand' its full meaning, complete with the speaker or writer's intent and sentiment."[9]

"Carbon-based units" (we humans) pose real challenges to the silicon-based machines that try to decipher the many inconsistencies we call language. Digital assistants like Alexa and Siri rely on their ability to convert speech into text, a process that uses NLP. Similarly, online services that translate English into many other human languages use NLP to tag words grammatically to determine whether they're verbs, nouns, or other parts of speech. NLP also performs word sense disambiguation, that is, determining the correct meaning of a word based on its context (e.g., "make" as a noun in a sentence describing a car versus in a sentence describing how to "make" bread). NLP can also perform sentiment analysis, which helps to identify the speaker's attitudes and emotions by evaluating the text spoken.

KEY TAKEAWAYS

- The capabilities of AI can surpass the ability of humans to diagnose disease, such as in detecting heart rhythm changes in ECGs.

- AI has the potential to increase accessibility to emerging healthcare by bringing specialized diagnostic tools to people who don't live near a large medical center.

- To build the digital solutions needed to transform healthcare, we first need a network of patient content that's safe, accurate, and unbiased. That's why Mayo Clinic Platform developed Mayo Clinic Platform_Connect.

References

|1| Noseworthy P, Attia A, Behnken E, et al. Artificial intelligence-guided screening for atrial fibrillation using electrocardiogram during sinus rhythm: A prospective non-randomised interventional trial. *Lancet.* 2022;400(10359):1206-1212. doi: 10.1016/S0140-6736(22)01637-3.

|2| Graham DJ, Campen D, Hui R, et al. Risk of acute myocardial infarction and sudden cardiac death in patients treated with cyclo-oxygenase 2 selective and nonselective non-steroidal anti-inflammatory drugs: Nested case-control study. *Lancet.* 2005;365(9458):475-581. doi: 10.1016/S01460-6736(05)17864-7.

|3| Graham D. Government Accountability Project. May 8, 2020. Accessed June 21, 2024. https://whistleblower.org/whistleblower-profiles/dr-david-graham/.

|4| Cerrato P, Halamka J. *Realizing the Promise of Precision Medicine.* Elsevier/Academic Press; 2018.

|5| Rieke, N. What is federated learning? Nvidia blog. October 13, 2019. Accessed November 5, 2024. https://blogs.nvidia.com/blog/what-is-federated-learning/.

|6| Murugadoss K, Rajasekharan A, Malin B, et al. Building a best-in-class automated de-identification tool for electronic health records through ensemble learning. *Patterns.* 2021;2(6) 100255. https://doi.org/10.1016/j.patter.2021.100255.

|7| Upadhyay S. What is an algorithm? Definition, Types, Characteristics. Simplilearn. October 17, 2023. Accessed December 11, 2023. https://www.simplilearn.com/tutorials/data-structure-tutorial/what-is-an-algorithm.

|8| Cerrato P, Halamka J. *Redefining the Boundaries of Medicine.* Mayo Clinic Press; 2023.

|9| IBM. What is NLP (natural language processing)? Accessed December 12, 2023. https://www.ibm.com/topics/natural-language-processing.

CHAPTER 2

Inventing the algorithms that transform healthcare

Ken Counihan lives an active lifestyle, using a smartwatch to monitor his workouts, count calories, and play music.[1] He never imagined it would also play a critical role in saving his life. Ken's smartwatch can track respirations, and he recently noticed that his number of breaths per minute had jumped from 14 to 17 or 18. It later informed him that his blood oxygen, which is normally 95 or higher, had dropped to the mid-80s. A trip to the emergency department at Ken's local hospital and additional tests revealed blood clots in his lungs—a life-threatening condition called pulmonary embolism! Fortunately, with smartwatch alerts, prompt medical follow-up, and the help of blood-thinning medications (anticoagulants), Ken's condition was stabilized.

Most casual observers who hear stories like Ken's rarely think about what's "under the hood," that is, the kinds of computer programs that make such discoveries possible. Chief among them are the algorithms we discussed in Chapter 1. We talked about creating a network containing data from millions of de-identified patient records, a source of new insights about what causes specific diseases and how to prevent and treat them. With that treasure trove of rich data in hand, the next logical step is to use it to develop digital tools to transform patient care—algorithms. As we explained in Chapter 1, an algorithm is a set of instructions that tell a computer how to perform a specific task. Put another way, it's a flowchart or roadmap with several forks in the road that invite you to go left or right, depending on the situation at hand. The eventual result is an "output," which in digital health might be a determination that a certain mole is benign or malignant, for example.

To most people, algorithms may not sound like an exciting topic, but understanding how they're built will make you a better consumer of online services and reduce the risk that you'll be duped into buying useless digital snake oil. If you're a patient, the knowledge will improve your interaction with the healthcare system and your ability to use the latest remote patient monitoring devices to your advantage.

Getting back to Ken's case history, blood oxygen level refers to the percentage of oxygen that red blood cells transport to tissues in the body, also called oxygen saturation. Typically, blood oxygen is measured at a doctor's office using a pulse oximeter, a small device that's clipped onto your fingertip. Some smartwatches can serve as pulse oximeters if they're loaded with a specific app.

Let's take a closer look at a blood oxygen app. There's a sensor on the back of the watch crystal that detects light. The light emitted by the sensor penetrates a person's skin to detect color changes in their blood. When blood is fully saturated with oxygen, it's bright red, but as it loses oxygen, it turns dark brown. With the help of a specially trained algorithm, those color changes can be analyzed to determine whether a person's oxygen saturation falls within the normal range.

HOW DO YOU BUILD A MEDICAL ALGORITHM?

Algorithms are everywhere, from your favorite streaming service to your bank's online systems, your credit card company's customer service department, and the antiviral software on your computer. If you subscribe to Netflix or a similar service, you've probably noticed that it suggests movies you might enjoy based on your previous choices. Sophisticated software programs are behind those recommendations. Sometimes, Netflix's algorithm can predict your taste, and sometimes it's completely off. Unfortunately, there's no place for that kind of poor performance in healthcare. Guessing wrong about what movie you'll like may annoy you, but predicting that you have little chance of developing breast cancer in the next 5 years when, in fact, your risk is high, obviously can have dire consequences. That's why technologists who develop medical algorithms must meet a higher standard.

To understand the steps that technologists follow to create algorithms—also called models—it would help to first get to know the different types of artificial intelligence (AI) that serve as the foundation for the models. These days, most algorithms are created using machine learning, a form of AI that enables software to learn from scanning tens of thousands of pieces of data. For example, a model designed to detect retinopathy, the eye disease that often complicates diabetes, would scan 10,000+ retinal images to identify unique features that characterize the disease. That includes changes in the appearance of the capillaries at the back of the eye and exudates, fluid that leaks from the blood vessels.

Once the algorithm had sampled enough retinal images, it would create a profile of what the eyes of a typical patient with diabetic retinopathy look like. If that profile generates an algorithm that's more accurate at detecting the disease than an expert eye specialist doing an eye exam, then the algorithm could be put into routine medical practice. However, if the algorithm fell short, the developers would use a process called back propagation to correct the mistakes and improve its detection rate. Algorithms to screen for diabetic eye disease are already available to patients.[2] There are also algorithms available to help screen for skin cancer and abnormal heart rhythms.

AI-FUELED ALGORITHMS IMPACT HEALTHCARE

Algorithms to help detect diabetic eye disease are only the tip of the digital health iceberg. Models to detect mental depression and pancreatic, brain, and breast cancer also show promise. Consider the research about brain tumors.

If you or someone you know has ever been suspected of having a brain tumor, you may be aware of the steps that may be required to determine if such a tumor is cancerous or benign. In some cases, a surgeon biopsies the mass and decides during the procedure what to do next. Typically, the surgeon takes a tissue sample and sends it to a laboratory, where it's processed, put on a slide, and analyzed by a pathologist. The analysis is time-consuming and often interferes with treatment. It would be ideal if the surgeon could know almost immediately whether the mass is malignant so that they can take appropriate therapeutic steps. With the assistance of a type of algorithm called a convolutional neural network (CNN), researchers at the

University of Michigan found a way to speed up the process of diagnosing a brain tumor. Using CNN, Dr. Todd Hollon and his colleagues were able to "predict brain tumor diagnosis in the operating room in under 150 seconds."[3] It takes 20 to 30 minutes, and in some cases, it can be days before a definitive diagnosis is available from a pathologist. Hollon and colleagues conducted a carefully controlled experiment to compare assessments of 278 specimens by CNN and human pathologists. They demonstrated that the interpretations by algorithm (along with specialized hardware) were just as accurate as those made by the pathologists (94.6% versus 93.9%).

CNNs are artificial neural networks (ANNs) and were given that name because in some ways, they mimic the function of the human nervous system with its neurons, axons, and dendrites. Data scientists like to compare neurons to the nodes that exist in an ANN. Data are input from a source—an image of the eye's retina, for instance—and fed into the first layer of nodes, as was shown in Chapter 1, Figure 1.2. Gradually, the neural network identifies the most important features of the image, which enables the algorithm to tell the difference between a normal retina and one that's diseased. In the case of a CNN, the process is somewhat different. As TechTarget explains it:

> ❝ The process starts by sliding a filter designed to detect certain features over the input image, a process known as the convolution operation (hence the name 'convolutional neural network'). The result of this process is a feature map that highlights the presence of the detected features in the image. The map then serves as input for the next layer, enabling a CNN to gradually build a hierarchical representation of the image. Initial filters usually detect basic features, such as lines or simple textures. The filters in subsequent layers are more complex, combining the basic features identified earlier on to recognize more complex patterns. For example, after an initial layer detects the presence of edges, a deeper layer could use that information to start identifying shapes."[4]

Hollon isn't the only medical scientist developing algorithms to improve diagnosis and treatment of brain tumors. Dutch surgeons and data scientists have devised a model using ANNs to identify additional abnormalities in tissue samples removed during brain surgery. The model detects changes in DNA referred to as methylation, which "provide a 'fingerprint' for each individual tumour and might match the methylation patterns of other tumours that behave in a similar way. Using a methylation classifier and machine learning approaches, an algorithm can compare the DNA-methylation profile of a tumour with a reference set of patterns for different tumour subtypes."[5] The information from the algorithm can help surgeons determine how much of a mass to take out while a patient is still on the operating table to ensure the best outcome. Depending on the type of tumor being removed, taking out too little could result in a poorer prognosis, whereas taking out too much would risk neurological complications.

The Dutch researchers used a procedure called nanopore DNA sequencing to detect the anomalies and a machine learning algorithm they called Sturgeon. A retrospective analysis showed that, in most cases, the model correctly diagnosed the tumor within 40 minutes. When they applied the technique in a clinical trial (a prospective study), Sturgeon correctly classified the tumors in 72% of patients in less than 45 minutes.

Technologists have also made major strides in diagnosing and treating colorectal cancer.

One gastroenterology journal stated: "It is now too conservative to suggest that CADe [computer-assisted detection] and CADx [computer-assisted diagnosis] carry the potential to revolutionize colonoscopy. The AI revolution has already begun."[6] Made in 2017, that statement has been amplified by more recent studies. Such evidence-based optimism is supported by results from active research, including the ability of new algorithms to accurately evaluate the inner lining of the colon and detect precancerous polyps.[7]

Improving detection of colon polyps starts with a metric called the adenoma detection rate (ADR), which refers to the percentage of patients who have one or more adenomas—a type of noncancerous tumor—that are identified during a screening colonoscopy. Clinical guidelines recommend an ADR of at least 25% in patients at average risk for colorectal cancer. Tactics to increase that rate have met with little success, but a computer-assisted system called EM-Automated-RT has proven effective in three ways. First, it improves a gastroenterologist's ability to differentiate between informative and blurry video frames in real time during a colonoscopy. Second, it helps the physician better detect debris, including residual stool. Finally, it improves inspection of the mucosal membrane lining the colon by dividing the video view into quadrants. A pilot study found that EM-Automated-RT produced a "significant increase in the mean mucosal visualization score, the average debris removal score, the average bowel distension score, and the average withdrawal time."[6]

Polyps are sometimes difficult to detect, especially if they're small or flat, or if their color is only slightly different from surrounding tissue. Approximately 22% of all polyps are missed, but a CADe system called Polyp-Alert uses AI algorithms to improve detection of polyp edges by analyzing every third frame in colonoscopy videos. One study found it could detect 98% of polyps in 61 randomly selected colonoscopies.[8]

More recent advances in AI-assisted gastroenterology include the work at Mayo Clinic. Gastroenterology is one of the specialties that has shown the most promise in terms of its application of AI and machine learning. For example, Mayo Clinic's Endoscopy Center is utilizing Mayo Clinic Platform's resources to explore the value of machine learning in gastroenterology with the assistance of ImaGine, a comprehensive library of endoscopic videos and images linked to clinical data about symptoms and diagnoses and from pathology and radiology reports. Also included are unedited full-length videos as well as video summaries of procedures that capture landmarks, specific abnormalities, and anatomical identifiers.

One of the problems with many of the studies supporting AI-based algorithms is their retrospective design, that is, they look backward in time to analyze patients who have already been treated. Retrospective studies are more likely to be flawed because sometimes, important details are left out of historical records. However, in the field of CADe, at least 10 prospective studies have been done, all of which were randomized controlled trials (RCTs). Because prospective studies look forward in time, they can be designed to include all the relevant details needed to arrive at a more precise conclusion. Most of the current evidence indicates that CADe is superior to standard colonoscopy, decreasing the likelihood that adenomas will be missed and increasing the likelihood that they'll be found. Several companies now make software as a medical device (SaMD) systems that improve miss and detection rates. The SaMD receives a digital signal from an endoscopy processor and then "outputs a graphical user interface featuring a bounding box at the coordinates of the potential polyp in real time on the existing procedure monitor."[9] In plain English, that means that as an endoscopist looks at a patient's colon on a computer screen, they also see a box around a suspicious lesion, which focuses their attention on that specific area. The endoscopist then can decide whether what they're seeing is really an adenoma or the signal from the SaMD was a false alarm.

Michael Wallace, MD, chief of the Division of Gastroenterology and Hepatology at Sheikh Shakhbout Medical City, Abu Dhabi, UAE, and a Professor of Medicine at Mayo Clinic, recently spearheaded a clinical research project that demonstrated the value of AI in colonoscopy.[10] He and his colleagues enrolled 230 patients in a randomized trial in which all the patients had two colonoscopies—one with AI and one without—on the same day. In one half of the group, the first colonoscopy was done with the aid of AI for diagnosis, and it wasn't used in the second colonoscopy. In the other half of the group, the order was reversed. The adenoma miss rate was only 15.5% in the patients who had an AI-assisted colonoscopy first, compared with 32.4% when the first procedure didn't benefit from the use of AI. Wallace and colleagues also reported false-negative rates of 6.8% versus 29.6% in the AI and non-AI groups, respectively. They concluded: "AI resulted in an approximately 2-fold reduction in miss rate of colorectal neoplasia, supporting AI-benefit in reducing perceptual errors for small and subtle lesions at standard colonoscopy." The AI-based system used in the experiment, GI Genius, relied on a CNN that was previously trained on over 2,600 polyps that were confirmed histologically. In 2021, the U.S. Food and Drug Administration approved GI Genius to assist clinicians in detecting colon lesions in real time during colonoscopy.

Studies like the one by Wallace and colleagues rely on advances in image analysis, but other types of AI are available to assist clinicians in identifying patients at risk for colon cancer. One innovative tool has been developed by Medial EarlySign, an Israeli company that uses readily available clinical parameters to determine a patient's risk of colorectal cancer. ColonFlag has been evaluated in a study of data from more than 17,000 Kaiser Permanente Northwest patients, including their ages, genders, and complete blood counts.[11] Nine hundred of the patients already had colorectal cancer. The result was a risk score that could be used to gauge the likelihood that the patients without colorectal cancer would go on to develop the disease. The researchers compared ColonFlag's ability to predict cancer with that derived from looking at low hemoglobin (Hgb) levels. (Hgb is a protein in red blood cells and its levels fall when colorectal cancer causes gastrointestinal bleeding.) ColonFlag was 34% better at identifying colorectal cancer within a 180-to-360-day period than low Hgb levels in patients between 50 and 75 years of age. The algorithm was more sensitive for detecting tumors in the cecum and ascending colon than in the transverse and sigmoid colon and rectum.

Mayo Clinic has developed a tool to help detect atrial fibrillation (an abnormal heart rhythm) and asymptomatic left ventricular systolic dysfunction, or ALVSD (an indication that a patient has a weak heart pump). That digital tool is partially based on an algorithm that was validated in patients during a controlled clinical trial called the EAGLE study. While ALVSD isn't the most well-known medical disorder, it increases a patient's risk of heart failure and death. Unfortunately, ALVSD isn't that easy to detect. Characterized by low ejection fraction (EF)—a measure of how much blood the heart pumps out during each contraction—ALVSD can be diagnosed with an echocardiogram. But because echocardiograms are expensive, they're not recommended for routinely screening the general public. The AI-enhanced algorithm, which

Figure 2.1 is a roadmap illustrating one approach to developing a health-care algorithm that relies on artificial intelligence. In Chapter 1, we discussed Steps 1 and 2. In this chapter, we briefly described the process of validating the algorithm. But as the graphic shows, there are two parts to this validation process.

During the creation of an algorithm, developers typically divide the collected samples into groups. Fifty percent to 70% of the images are used to train the model and 30% to 50% are used to test it.

If the goal were to identify melanoma, you might start with 10,000 skin samples and divide them into two groups. Group 1 would contain 5,000 images used to train a model that distinguishes cancer from normal models. The images would be tagged so that the model would know which was which and learn the features of cancer versus those of a mole. Group 2 also would contain 5,000 images, which would be used to test or validate the training. In our example, the model would be shown the images but not told which are cancer and which are not cancer. In such a case, validation refers to the ability to correctly classify a lesion without the help of a tag. That's called internal validation.

It's also important to perform external validation to make sure that an algorithm can be used on patients who were not part of the initial dataset. For instance, if the dataset included only patients from a clinic in rural Arkansas, results with it might not be useful for patients in New York City. In other words, the findings might not be generalizable. External validation typically includes studies of diverse patient populations and relies more on prospective data than on retrospective data.

Once a model has been validated internally and externally, the developer typically refines it based on feedback from those tests. Then it's launched in a real-world setting and its use is monitored over time to see how the tool performs.

FIGURE 2.1
How to develop a healthcare AI-driven algorithm

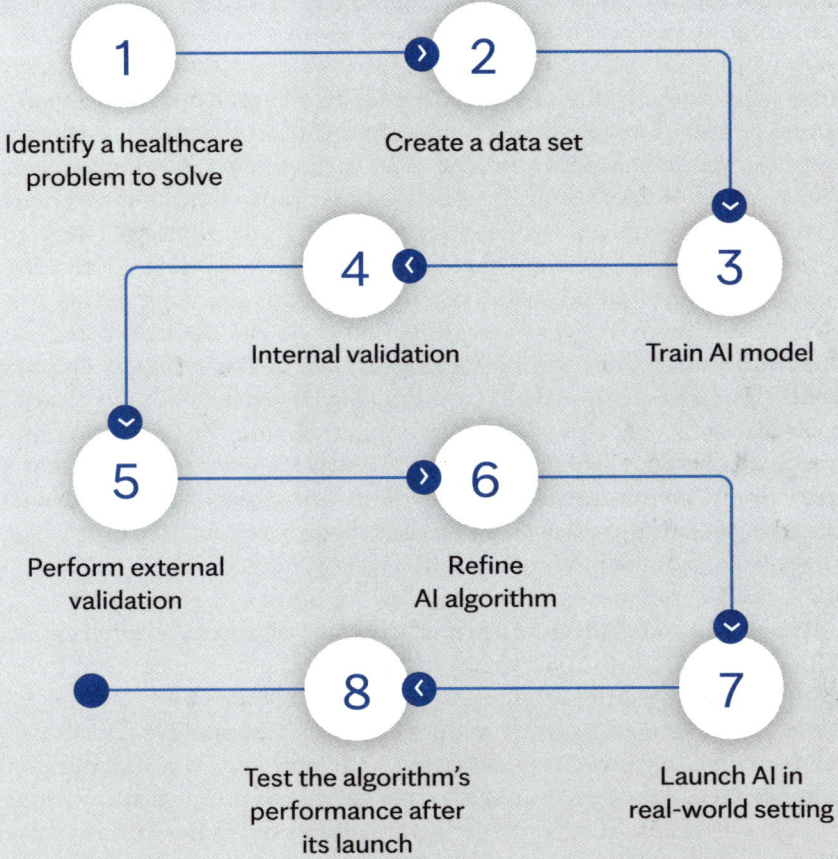

1 Identify a healthcare problem to solve

2 Create a data set

3 Train AI model

4 Internal validation

5 Perform external validation

6 Refine AI algorithm

7 Launch AI in real-world setting

8 Test the algorithm's performance after its launch

is used in conjunction with a routine electrocardiogram (ECG), can identify low EF. It's one of many advances that will eventually make AI an essential part of every clinician's "tool kit."

A collaborative effort by several of Mayo Clinic's clinical departments and Mayo Clinic Platform, the new algorithm, known as AI-ECG, was published as part of the EAGLE trial.[12] The trial included over 22,000 patients, who were divided into intervention and control groups and managed by 358 clinicians from 45 clinics and hospitals. AI-ECG was used to evaluate patients in both groups, but only clinicians who participated in the intervention arm had access to the AI results when they were deciding whether to order an echocardiogram. In the final analysis, 49.6% of patients whose physicians had access to the AI data received an echocardiogram, compared with only 38.1% whose physicians did not have access to the AI data. Xiaoxi Yao, with the Kern Center for the Science of Health Care Delivery, Mayo Clinic, and colleagues reported that "the intervention increased the diagnosis of low EF in the overall cohort (1.6% in the control arm versus 2.1% in the intervention arm) and among those who were identified as having a high likelihood of low EF." Using AI-ECG enabled primary care physicians to increase the diagnosis of low EF overall by 32% when compared with the rate in patients who received the usual care. In absolute terms, for every 1,000 patients screened, the AI system generated five new diagnoses of low EF compared with usual care. Earlier research on the neural network used to create the AI tool showed that it was supported by strong evidence.

More and more thought leaders in medicine are questioning the rush to generate AI-based algorithms because many lack the solid scientific foundation required to justify their use in direct patient care. Among the criticisms being leveled at AI developers are concerns about algorithms derived from a dataset that isn't validated with a second, external dataset, overreliance on retrospective analysis, lack of generalizability, and various types of bias. The EAGLE trial investigators addressed many of these concerns by testing their algorithm on more than one patient population. In an earlier study, the tool was used on over 44,000 Mayo Clinic patients to train the neural network and then tested on a second, independent group of nearly 53,000 patients. Although that research was retrospective, other prospective studies have confirmed the algorithm's value in clinical practice. The EAGLE trial was both prospective and pragmatic, meaning that it reflected the real world in which clinicians practice. Traditional RCTs consume a lot of resources, take a long time to conduct, and usually include a long list of criteria that are used to qualify patients or exclude them from participating. The EAGLE trial, on the other hand, was performed among patients in everyday practice.

KEY TAKEAWAYS

- Algorithms are the key ingredient used to digitally transform health. They are helping detect medical conditions such as depression, pancreatic and colon cancers, and brain tumors, just to name a few.

- A number of predictive artificial intelligence techniques are being used to improve the diagnoses of many life-threatening disorders.

- While digital tools are already helping many doctors provide better care, they are not a panacea. Some fall short because they aren't fully tested.

References

|1| Justice C. 'It saved my life': Cleveland man credits Apple Watch for life-saving medical discovery. News 5 Cleveland. March 16, 2023. Accessed January 22, 2024. https://www.news5cleveland.com/news/local-news/it-saved-my-life-cleveland-man-credits-apple-watch-for-life-saving-medical-discovery.

|2| Digital Diagnostics. LumineticsCore™. Accessed January 23, 2024. https://www.digitaldiagnostics.com/products/eye-disease/lumineticscore/.

|3| Hollon TC, Pandian B, Adapa AR, et al. Near real-time intraoperative brain tumor diagnosis using stimulated Raman histology and deep neural networks. *Nature Med.* 2020;26:52-58. doi: 10.1038/s41591-019-0715-9.

|4| Craig L. Convolutional neural network (CNN). Tech Accelerator. Accessed January 31, 2024. https://www.techtarget.com/searchenterpriseai/definition/convolutional-neural-network#:~:text=CNNs%20use%20a%20series%20of,layers%20to%20recognize%20detailed%20patterns.

|5| Baird LC. AI rapidly diagnoses brain tumours during surgery. *Nature.* 2023;622(7984):702-703. doi: 10.1038/d41586-023-03072-9.

|6| Byrne MF, Shahidi N, Rex DK. Will computer-aided detection and diagnosis revolutionize colonoscopy? *Gastroenterology.* 2017;153(6):1460-1464.E1.

| 7 | Cerrato P, Halamka J. *Reinventing Clinical Decision Support: Data Analytics, Artificial Intelligence, and Diagnostic Reasoning (HIMSS Book Series).* First Edition. Taylor & Francis; 2019.

| 8 | Wang Y, Tavanapong W, Won J, Oh JH, de Groen PC. Polyp-Alert: Near real-time feedback during colonoscopy. *Comput Methods Programs Biomed.* 2015;120(3):164-179. https://doi.org/10.1016/j.cmpb.2015.04.002.

| 9 | Shaukat A, Thompson R, et al. Computer-aided detection improves adenomas per colonoscopy for screening and surveillance colonoscopy: A randomized trial. *Gastroenterology.* 163(3): 732-741, quoted in Halamka J, Cerrato P. Computer-assisted diagnosis brings gastroenterology into the future. Mayo Clinic Platform (blog), https://www.mayoclinicplatform.org/2022/10/27 /computer-assisted-diagnosis-brings-gastroenterology-into-the-future/

| 10 | Wallace M, Sharma P, et al. Impact of artificial intelligence on miss rate of colorectal neoplasia. *Gastroenterology.* 2022;163(1):295-304.e5. https://doi.org /10.1053/j.gastro.2022.03.007.

| 11 | Hornbrook MC, Goshen R, Choman E, et al. Early colorectal cancer detected by machine learning model using gender, age, and complete blood count data. *Digest Dis Sci.* 2017;62(10): 2719-2727.

| 12 | Yao X, Rushlow DR, Inselman JW, et al. Artificial intelligence–enabled electro-cardiograms for identification of patients with low ejection fraction: A pragmatic, randomized clinical trial. *Nature Med.* 2021;27(5):815-819. doi: 10.1038 /s41591-021-01335-4.

CHAPTER 3

Keeping digital health safe and secure

In the Introduction and Chapters 1 and 2, we emphasized the positive impact that artificial intelligence (AI) and other internet-enabled tools are having on patients' health. But we can't ignore the dangers of some online content and apps. One critique of the internet states that it has "become a mortally polluted ocean of toxicity." More specifically, "The internet complex is the implacable engine of addiction, loneliness, false hopes, cruelty, indebtedness, psychosis, squandered life, the corrosion of memory, and social disintegration."[1] Obviously, this perspective presents only one side of the story. Online content also includes free access to a massive database of credible medical information in PubMed, enables many respected healthcare systems to dispense practical patient education materials, provides how-to videos to fix your plumbing problems, and much more. Given these contrasting views, we need safeguards to keep digital health content safe, secure, and effective.

EXPANDING THE DEFINITION OF DIGITAL HEALTH

Traditionally, digital health has been defined as "the use of information and communications technologies in medicine and other health professions to manage illnesses and health risks and to promote wellness."[2] The National Library of Medicine also explains that digital health has a broad scope and includes the use of wearable devices, mobile health, telehealth, health information technology, and telemedicine. The goals are to:

- Improve access to healthcare
- Reduce any inefficiencies in the healthcare system
- Improve the quality of care
- Lower the cost of healthcare
- Provide more personalized healthcare for patients

Subcategories of digital health include:

- Remote sensing and wearables
- Telemedicine and health information
- Data analytics and intelligence, predictive modeling
- Health and wellness behavior modification tools
- Bioinformatics tools
- Medical social media
- Digitized health record platforms
- Patient-physician portals
- Do-it-yourself diagnostics, compliance, and treatments
- Decision support systems
- Imaging

The emphasis in digital health has always been on what healthcare professionals can do to improve patient well-being. In the future, digital health experts will also need to take a critical look at the impact that the internet, including social media sites, is having on people's mental health. That's a major concern for anyone who cares for teenagers and young adults.[3]

Many experts have documented evidence of a mental health crisis among the young. The American Psychological Association points out: "The COVID-19 pandemic era ushered in a new set of challenges for youth in the United States, leading to a mental health crisis as declared by the United States surgeon general just over a year ago. But U.S. children and teens have been suffering for far longer. In the 10 years leading up to the pandemic, feelings of persistent sadness and hopelessness—as well as suicidal thoughts and behaviors—increased by about 40% among young people, according to the Centers for Disease Control and Prevention's (CDC) Youth Risk Behavior Surveillance System."[4] By one estimate, about 17 million children in the United States will experience a mental health disorder by the time they reach age 18.[5] The effects of social media on adolescent mental health are complex, but Richard Horton, MD, editor of *The Lancet,* believes the crisis is "fueled by the greed of internet entrepreneurs who see children as objects for manipulation and profit."[1] That might be an overstatement, but there is evidence to indicate that unscrupulous promotion of social media content is having a detrimental effect on impressionable minds.

In a 2023 advisory, *Social Media and Youth Mental Health,*[6] the U.S. Surgeon General's Office noted that up to 95% of individuals ages 13 to 17 use a social media platform, more than one-third of whom do so "almost constantly." The advisory further points out that the effect of social media on individual children and adolescents varies, depending on their unique strengths and vulnerabilities, as well as cultural, historical, and socioeconomic factors. There is broad agreement among the scientific community that social media has the potential to both benefit and harm children and adolescents. One study found that teens who spent more than 3 hours a day on social media were twice as likely to have mental health problems, including symptoms of depression and anxiety.[7] Of course, just because social media is associated with psychiatric conditions doesn't prove that it *contributes* to depression and anxiety. It's also possible that teenagers who are already depressed and anxious gravitate to social media to help cope with their emotional problems.

Nonetheless, the link between social media and adolescent mental health does raise concerns about its potential harm. In a unique natural experiment that leveraged the staggered introduction of a social media platform across U.S. colleges, the rollout of the platform was associated with an increase in depression (9% over baseline) and anxiety (12% over baseline) among college-age youth (359,827 observations were taken into consideration).[8] The study's co-author also noted that had it been applied across the entirety of the U.S. college population, introduction of the platform would have contributed to more than 300,000 new cases of depression. If, in fact, such sizable effects have occurred in college-age youth, those findings would raise serious concerns about the risk of harm to children and adolescents who are exposed to social media at an even more vulnerable stage of brain development.

If excess use of social media really is causing a mental health problem among young people, limiting exposure to it might be expected to have a positive impact. The surgeon general's advisory suggests that's the case: A small randomized controlled trial (RCT) in college-age youth found that limiting social media use to 30 minutes a day over 3 weeks significantly reduced the severity of depression—from an average reading of 23 on the Beck Depression Inventory to 14.5 in 4 weeks.[6] The effect was most pronounced among individuals with high baseline levels of depression, in whom depression scores improved by more than 35%. Another RCT in young adults and adults found that deactivating a social media platform for 4 weeks improved subjective well-being (i.e., self-reported happiness, life satisfaction, depression, and anxiety) by 25%-40% of the effect of psychological interventions such as self-help therapy, group training, and individual therapy.[9]

Exactly how do certain types of social media harm the developing brains of teens? Sampling online content tells a disturbing story. Some social media sites feature live depictions of self-destructive acts such as partial asphyxiation and cutting and individuals talking about making suicide pacts. Many sites encourage disordered eating and unrealistic body image. And approximately 64% of teens are often or sometimes exposed to hate-based content on social media.[10] The list of harmful content goes on and on, prompting many stakeholders to call for better policies and more government regulation of social media platforms.

A detailed discussion of the social media problem is beyond the scope of our book, but we have provided a summary of the recommendations made by the U.S. Department of Health and Human Services to fix the problems. The agency's guidance for safe social media development and use includes the following:[6]

- Strengthen protections to ensure greater safety for children interacting with all social media platforms, in collaboration with governments, academic organizations, public health experts, and technology companies.

- Develop age-appropriate health and safety standards for technology platforms. Such standards may include designing technology that is appropriate and safe for a child's developmental stage; protecting children and adolescents from accessing harmful content (e.g., content that encourages eating disorders, violence, substance abuse, sexual exploitation, and suicide or discusses suicide means); limiting the use of features that attempt to maximize time, attention, and engagement; developing tools that protect activities that are essential for healthy development, like sleep; and regularly assessing and mitigating risks to children and adolescents.

- Require a higher standard of data privacy for children to protect them from potential harms like exploitation and abuse. Sixty percent of adolescents say they think they have little or no control over the personal information that social media companies collect about them.

- Pursue policies that further limit access to social media for all children—in ways that minimize the risk of harm—including strengthening and enforcing age minimums. Ensure technology companies share data relevant to the health impact of their platforms with independent researchers and the public in a manner that's timely, sufficiently detailed, and protects privacy.

- Support the development, implementation, and evaluation of digital and media literacy curricula in schools and as part of academic standards. Digital and media literacy provides children and educators with digital skills to strengthen digital resilience, or the ability to recognize, manage, and recover from online risks (e.g., cyberbullying and other forms of online harassment and abuse, and excessive use of social media).

- Support increased funding for future research about the benefits and harms of social media and other technology and digital media for children, adolescents, and families.

- Engage with international partners working to protect children and adolescents against online harm to their health and safety.

Equally important are recommendations directed at the technology companies that develop and host social media sites:[6]

- Conduct and facilitate transparent and independent assessments of the impact of social media products and services on children and adolescents. Assume responsibility for the impact of products on different subgroups and ages of children and adolescents, regardless of the intent behind them.

- Assess the potential risks of online interactions and take active steps to prevent potential misuse, reducing exposure to harms. When proactive responses fail, take immediate action to mitigate unintended negative effects.

- Establish scientific advisory committees to inform approaches and policies aimed at creating safe online environments for children. Scientific advisory committees should be composed of independent experts and members of user subgroups, including youth.

- Prioritize user health and safety in the design and development of social media products and services.

- Prioritize and leverage expertise in developmental psychology and user mental health and well-being in product teams to minimize risk of harm to children and adolescents.

- Ensure that default settings for children are set to the highest safety and privacy standards. Provide easy-to-read and highly visible information about policies regarding use by children.

- Adhere to and enforce age minimums in ways that respect the privacy of youth users.

- Design, develop, and evaluate platforms, products, and tools that foster safe and healthy online environments for youth, keeping in mind the needs of girls, racial, ethnic, and sexual and gender minorities. Platform design and algorithms should prioritize health and safety as the first principle, seek to maximize potential benefits, and avoid design features that attempt to maximize time, attention, and engagement.

- Share data about the health impact of the platforms and the strategies that are used to ensure safety and well-being with independent researchers and the public in a manner that's timely and protects privacy.

- Create effective and timely systems and processes to adjudicate requests and complaints from young people, families, educators, and others to address online abuse, harmful content and interactions, and other threats to children's health and safety. Social media platforms should take these complaints seriously, thoroughly investigate and consider them, and respond in a timely and transparent manner.

COALITION FOR HEALTH AI

As we mentioned earlier, digital health typically refers to the use of information and communication technologies to manage illnesses and health risks and to promote wellness. With that in mind, many clinicians and technologists have been working diligently to provide safe, secure, and accurate algorithms that improve patient care rather than hinder it.

You've probably never heard of a nonprescription medicine that was popular in the early 20th century called "Pink Pills for Pale People." Ads for the pills claimed that they cured nervous headaches, rheumatism, ataxia, palpitations, and pale complexion. Those claims were based on a kernel of truth because the pills contained iron sulfate, which would have relieved the pallor brought on by iron deficiency anemia. But like many other "miracle drugs" of that era, the scientific foundation upon which the Pink Pills rested wasn't very trustworthy. The same is true of many AI-based algorithms coming to market today.

Many digital tools don't solve the problems they were designed to address, or they do more harm than good. That's one of the reasons the Coalition for Health AI (CHAI) was created. CHAI is a community of academic health systems, organizations, and expert AI and data science practitioners, including Mayo Clinic. CHAI members came together to harmonize standards and reporting for health AI and to educate end users about how to evaluate the technologies to drive their adoption.

In 2023, CHAI published its *Blueprint for Trustworthy AI Implementation Guidance and Assurance for Healthcare* to build confidence in a set of principles that developers, healthcare providers, and other stakeholders can rely on.[11] Like all organizations involved in digital health, the Coalition is aware of the need to earn the trust of all its stakeholders. One way to accomplish that is to involve a wide variety of thought leaders from several segments of the healthcare ecosystem. That includes data scientists, software engineers, vendors, physicians, nurses, clinicians in training, insurers, patient advisory groups, government regulators, research funders, educators, and many others.

As the *Blueprint* points out:

66 This work has brought together a collaboration across a number of institutions with expertise in different areas relevant to this effort to attain sufficiently broad coverage. The goal is to ensure applicability to a wide range of clinical AI-based systems and thus facilitate more widespread adoption. Some of the institutions that have already published guidelines (i.e., Mayo Clinic, Duke, Stanford, Johns Hopkins) are part of this work. While there are current efforts to develop core ingredients for AI/ML [artificial intelligence/machine learning] for specific medical applications like cardiac software and medical devices, the clinical AI/ML community would benefit from an approach that could be applied to AI-based clinical algorithms for various uses (e.g., diagnostic, prognostic) and clinical subdomains (e.g., oncology, cardiology).

The document goes on to say that:

66 CHAI is playing an important role in validating AI algorithms, which is one of the primary reasons the organization was developed. But validation is only one part of the formula for reliable, safe algorithms.

We also realize that healthcare AI is a moving target, with new technologies rapidly emerging month by month. Thus, the need for "sandboxes" to test these emerging innovations, as well as assurance accreditation labs and technical assistance services. (In the world of technology, a sandbox is like a child's sandbox; in this safe digital space, developers can build and experiment with new tools without doing any damage in the real world. Put another way, it's "a system that allows an untrusted application to run in a highly controlled environment where the application's permissions are restricted to an essential set of computer permissions.")[11, 12]

The need for reliable, safe digital tools that can improve the diagnostic process and foster new treatment options has never been greater, and it's been recognized by technology companies and government officials. With these concerns in mind, in 2023, the White House issued an executive order on safe, secure, and trustworthy AI that's bound to impact developers, technology companies, and providers alike.[13] To protect the public from the potential risks of AI systems, the order requires:

- Developers of the most powerful AI systems to share their safety test results and other critical information with the U.S. government.

- Development of standards, tools, and tests to help ensure that AI systems are safe, secure, and trustworthy.

- Protection against the risks of using AI to engineer dangerous biological materials.

- Protection of Americans from AI-enabled fraud and deception by establishing standards and best practices for detecting AI-generated content and authenticating official content.

- Establishment of an advanced cybersecurity program to develop AI tools to find and fix vulnerabilities in critical software.

- Development of a National Security Memorandum that directs further actions on AI and security.

The new directive instructs the U.S. Department of Health and Human Services (HHS) to create a system that accepts reports from users about AI dangers and unsafe practices and to do something about the issues.[13] According to *Stat News,* the United States is behind the European Union (EU) in developing standards to provide guardrails for healthcare AI. In

March 2024, the EU adopted the Artificial Intelligence Act, which prohibits the following practices because they pose an unacceptable risk to public and individual safety:[14]

- The use of facial recognition technology in public places
- AI that may influence political campaigns
- Social scoring AI that classifies people based on certain characteristics or behaviors
- Emotion recognition AI

Offenders who violate these prohibitions can be fined up to €40 million (about $42 million).

The regulations enacted by the United States and Europe may not address all the challenges that have surfaced since the introduction of ChatGPT-4 and similar large language models. But they're an important step in the right direction. These regulations are consistent with the goals and objectives of CHAI, which hopes to energize a coalition of the willing to join them in their quest to earn the trust of all healthcare stakeholders.

The CHAI *Blueprint* lists several key elements required to create trustworthy healthcare AI, including the need for it to be useful, safe, accountable, transparent, explainable, and easily interpreted. In addition, the *Blueprint* emphasizes the importance of algorithms being fair, which means they must address systemic, computational, statistical, and cognitive biases. Equally important, CHAI states that these digital tools should be secure and protect user privacy. That's a tall order for any developer to meet, but the *Blueprint* provides detailed advice for doing so, which is beyond the scope of our book.

VALIDATING THE TOOLS THAT DRIVE DIGITAL HEALTH

In previous chapters, we mentioned the importance of validating algorithms. In the past, that hasn't always been a priority for the developers of digital health tools. In their rush to go to market with a salable product, some companies cut corners, and in the end, that only hurts patients and frustrates healthcare providers who are using the tools at the bedside. On the flip side, developers who do their due diligence stand out by "checking all the necessary boxes."

For example, in 2018, IDx-DR, a software system used to improve screening for retinopathy, became the first AI-based medical device to receive U.S. Food and Drug Administration (FDA) clearance to "detect greater than a mild level of . . . diabetic retinopathy in adults who have diabetes." (Retinopathy is a common complication of diabetes.)

To arrive at its decision about IDx-DR, the FDA not only reviewed data that established the system's safety but also took into account results from prospective studies, which are an essential type of evidence that clinicians look for when trying to decide if a device or product is worth using. IDx-DR is the first FDA-cleared medical device that doesn't require the services of a specialist to interpret the results, making it a useful tool for healthcare providers who aren't typically involved in eye care. The FDA clearance emphasized the fact that IDx-DR—now called LumineticsCore—is for screening and not diagnosis, and that patients with positive results should be referred to an eye care professional. The algorithm built into the IDx-DR system is intended to be used with the Topcon NW400 retinal camera and a cloud server that contains the software.

Similarly, the FDA reviewed results from a prospective randomized trial before approving GI Genius, a machine learning-based algorithm that can help endoscopists improve their ability to detect small, easily missed colon polyps. The agency's recent clearance of the Medtronic computer-aided detection (CADe) system was based on clinical trial results published in *Gastroenterology*. Investigators in Italy evaluated data from 685 patients and compared a group who underwent the procedure with the help of GI Genius to a group who acted as controls. Repici and colleagues found that the adenoma detection rate was significantly higher in the CADe group, as was the detection rate for polyps 5 mm or smaller, which led them to conclude that "including CADe in colonoscopy examinations increases detection of adenomas without affecting safety."[15]

The findings from the study of GI Genius raise several questions. Is it reasonable to assume that a study of 600+ Italians would apply to a U.S. population, which has different demographic characteristics? More importantly, were those 685 patients representative of the general public and did they include enough individuals of color and from lower socioeconomic groups? Although the report about the study in *Gastroenterology* did mention enough female patients, the authors said nothing about other groups that may be marginalized.

An independent 2021 analysis of FDA approvals also raised several concerns about the effectiveness and equity of other recently approved AI algorithms. Wu and colleagues at Stanford University examined FDA clearances of 130 devices and found that the vast majority of the approvals (126 of 130) were based on results from retrospective studies. And when the researchers separated all 130 devices into low- and high-risk subgroups using FDA guidelines, they found that none of the 54 high-risk devices had been evaluated in prospective trials.*[16] Other shortcomings of the reports documented in Wu's analysis included the following:

- Single-center rather than multicenter evaluation for 93 of the 130 approved products;

- No mention of sample size of the test population for 59 of the approved AI devices; and

- Mention of a demographic subgroup in studies of only 17 of the approved devices, which suggests that the researchers may have ignored often marginalized groups like people of color, women, and the poor.

At Mayo Clinic, we've spent years creating and refining the digital tools needed to validate healthcare algorithms. Mayo Clinic_Validate evaluates the bias, specificity, and sensitivity of AI models, enabling developers to provide a measure of assurance that their algorithm is accurate and unbiased. Because this validation process is conducted by an independent third party, it gives clinicians more confidence in a model's usefulness in clinical practice.

The "yardsticks" used to perform validation—sensitivity and specificity—may be unfamiliar to you if you don't have a background in statistics. Sensitivity refers to how accurately a tool pinpoints a condition in patients who have it. So, a model designed to detect skin cancer that has a sensitivity of 80% can correctly identify 80 of 100 patients who actually have the disease. Of course, that also implies that the remaining 20 patients who have skin cancer and are tested with the model will be told that they do not have the disease even though they do. Specificity refers to a model's ability to accurately identify patients who do not have the condition being tested for.

---

*Evidence from retrospective studies is much weaker than evidence from prospective studies because retrospective studies are based on data from the charts of past patients and important information may be missing from that documentation. Prospective studies are done in real time and take into account many of the confounding factors that can distort findings from retrospective studies.

A specificity rating of 90% means that 90 of 100 patients who test negative for the condition using a model do not have it.

ASSURANCE LABS PLAY A CRITICAL ROLE

Some entrepreneurs may object to all the effort being made to regulate and monitor the quality of AI algorithms. After all, the marketplace has a way of regulating itself through stiff competition. Higher-quality products and services thrive and poor performers fall by the wayside. That's fine for an algorithm that helps you choose movies to watch on Netflix or Amazon Prime, where the worst-case scenario is time wasted on a movie you don't like. In healthcare, however, the stakes are much higher. Life-threatening consequences are a distinct possibility if AI comes up short on a diagnosis.

A few years ago, a poorly performing medical algorithm made headlines. Epic Sepsis Model (ESM) was designed to help medical professionals predict the onset of sepsis, a life-threatening buildup of harmful microorganisms in the blood or other tissues. ESM was offered to clinicians as part of an electronic health record system developed by Epic and used on tens of thousands of inpatients after being tested by the vendor on over 400,000 patients in three health systems. Unfortunately, because ESM is a proprietary algorithm, little information is available about the software's inner workings or its long-term performance. Wong and colleagues at the University of Michigan conducted a detailed analysis of the tool among over 27,600 patients and found it wanting. One of the statistics used to evaluate the accuracy of the algorithm, called the area under the receiver operating characteristic curve (AUROC), was quite low, only 0.63. The authors' report states: "The ESM identified 183 of 2552 patients with sepsis (7%) who did not receive timely administration of antibiotics, highlighting the low sensitivity of the ESM in comparison with contemporary clinical practice. The ESM also did not identify 1709 patients with sepsis (67%) despite generating alerts for an ESM score of 6 or higher for 6971 of all 38,455 hospitalized patients (18%), thus creating a large burden of alert fatigue." Wong and colleagues went on to discuss the far-reaching implications of their investigation: "The increase and growth in deployment of proprietary models has led to an underbelly of confidential, non-peer-reviewed model performance documents that may not accurately reflect real-world model performance."[17]

Shortcomings like this have made many healthcare professionals and patients skeptical of AI. So, how do we get scientifically well-documented digital health tools into clinicians' hands and convince them and their patients that AI is trustworthy? One approach is to develop an evaluation system that impartially reviews all the specs for each product. That's the idea behind AI assurance labs.

Nigam Shah, MBBS, PhD, the chief data scientist for Stanford Health Care, and colleagues have explained how these labs would improve model accuracy and safety, and ultimately benefit patients.[18] A nationwide network of assurance labs offers several advantages. To begin with, these labs can spur development by companies interested in entering the marketplace, rather than slow it down, as some critics have suggested. The labs can act as a shared resource that can be tapped by developers with little expertise in healthcare to point them in the right direction. Healthcare professionals continue to complain about "an ecosystem dominated by well-meaning but often overexuberant and inexperienced developers who lack the depth of understanding of health care delivery."[18]

The labs would also enable developers to ensure that their products have undergone a comprehensive evaluation. That includes technical assessment of a model as well as bias analysis and usability testing. In addition, if the labs are designed correctly, they would be capable of simulating how an algorithm would perform in the real world, where it would be subject to all sorts of regulations, hospital policies, and *workflow* limitations. Too often, that last constraint is overlooked.

By way of analogy, consider the success of online stores hosted by Walmart or Amazon. These companies have invested heavily in state-of-the-art supply chains that ensure their products are available from warehouses as customers demand them. But without a delivery service that gets products into customers' homes quickly and with a minimum of disruption, even the best products will sit on warehouse shelves. The delivery service has to seamlessly integrate into customers' lives. The product has to show up on time, it has to be the right-size garment, in a sturdy box, and so on. Similarly, the best diagnostic and predictive algorithms have to be delivered with careful forethought and insight, which requires design thinking, process improvement, workflow integration, and implementation science.

Equally important, AI assurance labs, if made available to the public, will provide transparency, especially if reports are published in plain language so that patients and practitioners can make informed decisions about the worth of algorithms. The failed sepsis algorithm we mentioned earlier illustrates the need for such transparency: ESM was constructed using proprietary technology from Epic that was not available to independent investigators.

WE CAN'T OVERLOOK CYBERSECURITY

Patients can't benefit from all that digital health has to offer if their medical information doesn't remain private and secure. We've written extensively for professional audiences about the importance of protecting patient information, and most of that guidance also is relevant to patients and the general public as well.[19]

Anyone who picks up a newspaper or scans online news service headlines knows all too well how many threats there are to everyone's personal data. Large hospitals are regularly being hacked and their patient records are being blocked until they're forced to pay a hefty ransom. And ransom is only the tip of the iceberg. Patients and consumers are being bombarded with email scams, websites infected with malware, phone calls from impostors who claim to represent government agencies, and on and on.

Even before all these threats became part of our everyday lives, the U.S. government took steps to protect sensitive patient information by creating the Health Insurance Portability and Accountability Act (HIPAA) system. HIPAA is a federal law enacted in 1996 that required the creation of national standards to protect sensitive patient health information from being disclosed without a patient's consent or knowledge.

HHS issued the HIPAA Privacy Rule to implement the requirements of HIPAA. The Privacy Rule standards address the use and disclosure of individuals' health information (known as protected health information, or PHI) by entities subject to the Privacy Rule. These individuals and organizations are called covered entities. The entities include healthcare providers, insurance companies, healthcare clearinghouses, and business associates who work with any of these organizations.

The Privacy Rule also contains standards for individuals' rights to understand and control how their health information is used. A major goal of the Privacy Rule is to make sure that individuals' health information is properly protected while allowing the flow of health information needed to provide and promote high-quality healthcare, and to protect the public's health and well-being. The Privacy Rule permits important uses of information while protecting the privacy of people who seek care and healing.

While the HIPAA Privacy Rule safeguards PHI, the Security Rule[20] protects a subset of information covered by the Privacy Rule, called electronic PHI or e-PHI. This is all individually identifiable health information that a covered entity creates, receives, maintains, or transmits in electronic form. The Security Rule doesn't apply to PHI transmitted orally or in writing. To comply with the HIPAA Security Rule, the covered entities must:

- Ensure the confidentiality, integrity, and availability of all e-PHI.

- Detect and safeguard against anticipated threats to the security of the information.

- Protect against anticipated impermissible uses or disclosures that are not allowed by the rule.

- Certify compliance by their workforce.

Covered entities should rely on professional ethics and best judgment when considering requests for permissive uses and disclosures. The HHS Office for Civil Rights enforces HIPAA rules, and all complaints should be reported to that office. HIPAA violations may result in civil monetary or criminal penalties. Several organizations have been required to pay multimillion-dollar fines for violating the regulations.

On a more practical note, there are several steps that healthcare organizations and patients can take to reduce the risk of having their digital health information exposed, including encryption, strong passwords, firewalls, antimalware software, and basic cyber hygiene.

Encryption

Encryption is a way to disguise text or other information so it's not recognizable to others. This means converting characters in a message into gibberish so they can't be read by unauthorized individuals and having a way to decode or "decrypt" the message so it can be read by authorized individuals. To oversimplify the process, it involves turning the letters "a," "b," and "c" into "x," "j," and "q." (Technically speaking, this is a substitution cipher, which is encoding, not encryption.)

Unfortunately, simple substitution of one letter for another is far too easy for today's hackers to decode, so modern cryptographers use sophisticated algorithms and protect them with encryption and decryption keys that prevent others from deciphering patient data that are supposed to remain confidential.

The original patient information is referred to as plaintext and the encoded information is ciphertext (Figure. 3.1). The algorithm converts the plaintext to ciphertext, which is based on a set of rules that tell the computer how to translate between the plaintext and the encrypted messages. For example, if we were to look at a simple substitution cipher, the rule might call for the conversion of every letter to three letters later in the alphabet, thus substituting every "a" character to a "d," "b" to an "e," and so on.

Modern cryptographic algorithms are typically based on the use of keys. The encryption key serves as the mechanism to instruct the computer how to translate the ciphertext back into a plaintext message. These keys can use two alternatives. The first system, called symmetric encryption, requires a single key to encrypt and decrypt the message. A second system, referred to as a public key or asymmetric cryptography, makes use of a publicly available key for encryption and a separate private key for decrypting. It's considered more secure but takes longer and requires more processing power.

Modern cryptographic algorithms are based on very computationally difficult mathematical problems, and the strength of the security around the encrypted message can vary with the length of the key used when it was encrypted. Choosing a strong key is one of the factors in ensuring that the message is not decrypted by unauthorized parties.

FIGURE 3.1

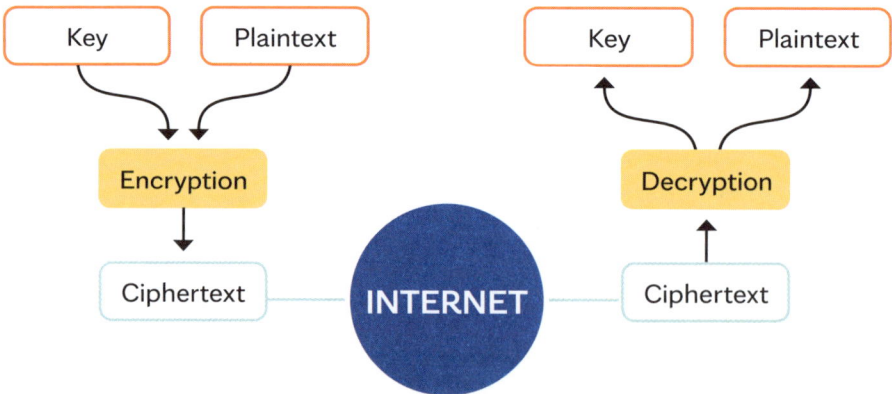

Firewalls

In the real world (that is, the one not composed of 0s and 1s), a firewall separates your car's engine compartment from the cabin, physically protecting it in case the engine bursts into flames. In cyberspace, firewalls have a similar function; they're hardware or software that serves as the first line of defense, offering a measure of protection by blocking suspicious traffic from the internet. They can also be placed inside an organization's network to shield sensitive information from unauthorized internal users.

On a personal computer, a firewall is typically built into a Netgear or Linksys router that sends data to your home network. If your computer also has an antimalware program by Norton, McAfee, or another vendor, there's probably also a firewall in that program. Someone running a medical practice, hospital, or other organization that handles PHI may want a deeper understanding of the types of firewalls available and where they are best positioned. In that case, the services of a skilled consultant may make sense.

Antimalware/antiviral software

Before you can make an intelligent decision about the type of antimalware program to invest in, it helps to understand what the term "malware" currently encompasses. In the broadest sense, malware is any type of software with malicious intent. That can range from theft of confidential patient information to disruption of your computer system's ability to function, destruction of data, or even locking up your data so that they can't be accessed by authorized users until you pay a ransom. In addition to viruses, your software should be able to detect Trojans, bots, worms, spyware, and rootkits. Here's a brief glossary of some of these infectious agents:

- A *digital virus,* similar to its biological counterpart, can copy itself once inside a computer and hide until the time is right to strike. Eventually the computer user takes some action that triggers the malware to do its mischief. Once the time bomb goes off, the malware delivers its "payload" and the user has to deal with the consequences. That may be an obscene sentence flashed across the screen or the machine's processing ability may slow down, or the malware may steal passwords.

- A *Trojan* derives its name from the fact that it looks like a normal file that has value to the user, tricking them into downloading it. Doing so can result in stolen data, modification of files, or keylogging, which enables outsiders to record every keystroke entered into the computer.

- Similarly, some *spyware* can track a user's activities and identify each keystroke as you type, which means it may be able to read your Social Security number, date of birth, and password as you type them on the keyboard.

- What makes *worms* so hideous is that, unlike a traditional virus, they don't need a human computer user to trigger them. A worm might attack your email list and send copies of itself to all your contacts.

When choosing an antimalware program, look for one that detects garden-variety viruses and other types of malware. Also make sure the software is installed on all your machines. Email servers should have email server antimalware software, workstations should have desktop protection, and servers should have programs designed to protect them.

Equally important is ensuring that these programs are set to automatically download regular updates. New malware shows up every day, so without updates, a protection program will be almost useless. That also means that if you disconnect from the internet for an extended period of time, your software will no longer be up to date because the program couldn't contact the antimalware company to look for the updates. When you install a new antimalware program, instruct the software to do regular scans of the machine.

While we're on the subject of updates, if you work in healthcare, someone in your office or department should be responsible for checking for updates to all your applications and your operating system. If Microsoft sends out a Windows update, it may contain a patch to plug a hole in the system that compromises security. Setting up Windows-based computers to get automatic updates is recommended. The same advice applies to anyone trying to keep their healthcare information secure on a personal computer.

The benefits of digital health are impressive, but when entering the online world, we can't ignore "the dark side of the Force."

KEY TAKEAWAYS

- Digital health has the potential to improve access to healthcare providers, provide greater personalized care, and reduce medical bills.

- To realize these benefits, digital health tools must come with "guard-rails," including government regulations and strong cybersecurity systems.

- Digital healthcare is a speeding train moving faster than anyone expected. Organizations like the Coalition for Health AI (CHAI) exist to keep the train from going off the rails.

References

|1| Horton R. Offline: The internet—A line has been crossed. *Lancet.* 2024;403: 600. https://www.thelancet.com/action/showPdf?pii=S0140-6736%2824%2900293-9.

|2| Ronquillo Y, Meyers A, Korvek SJ. Digital Health. [Updated 2023 May 1]. In: *StatPearls.* StatPearls Publishing; 2024. https://www.ncbi.nlm.nih.gov/books/NBK470260/.

|3| Anderer S. Social media industry standards needed to protect adolescent mental health, says National Academies. *JAMA.* 2024;331(7):552-553. doi: 10.1001/jama.2023.28259.

|4| Abrams Z. Kids' mental health is in crisis. Here's what psychologists are doing to help. American Psychological Association. January 1, 2023. Accessed August 22, 2024. https://www.apa.org/monitor/2023/01/trends-improving-youth-mental-health.

|5| Coe E. Getting to the bottom of the teen mental health crisis. *McKinsey Health Institute.* September 7, 2023. Accessed August 22, 2024. https://www.mckinsey.com/mhi/our-insights/getting-to-the-bottom-of-the-teen-mental-health-crisis.

|6| U.S. Surgeon General. *Social Media and Youth Mental Health.* 2023. Accessed August 22, 2024. https://www.hhs.gov/sites/default/files/sg-youth-mental-health-social-media-advisory.pdf.

|7| Riehm KE, Feder KA, Tormohlen KN, et al. Associations between time spent using social media and internalizing and externalizing problems among US youth. *JAMA Psychiatry.* 2019;76(12):1266-1273. doi.org/10.1001/jamapsychiatry.2019.2325.

| 8 | Braghieri L, Levy R, Makarin A. Social Media and Mental Health. *Amer Econ Rev.* 2022;112(11):3660-3693. https://pubs.aeaweb.org/doi/abs/10.1257/aer .20211218.

| 9 | Allcott H, Braghieri L, Eichmeyer S, Gentzkow M. The Welfare Effects of Social Media. *Am Econ Rev.* 2020;110(3):629-676. doi: 10.1257/aer.20190658.

| 10 | Rideout V, Robb MB. Social media, social life: Teens reveal their experiences. Common Sense Media, 2018. Accessed August 22, 2024. https://www.common sensemedia.org/sites/default/files/research/report/2018-social-media-social -life-executive-summary-web.pdf.

| 11 | Coalition for Health AI. *Blueprint for Trustworthy AI Implementation Guidance and Assurance for Healthcare Version 1.0.* April 4, 2023. Accessed August 22, 2024. https://chai.org/wp-content/uploads/2024/05/blueprint-for-trustworthy -ai_V1.0-2.pdf.

| 12 | NIST Computer Security Resource Center. Sandbox. Accessed April 2, 2024. https://csrc.nist.gov/glossary/term/sandbox#:~:text=Definitions%3A,file%20 system%20or%20the%20network.

| 13 | The White House. FACT SHEET: Biden-Harris administration executive order directs DHS to lead the responsible development of artificial intelligence. October 30, 2023. Accessed April 3, 2024. https://www.dhs.gov/archive /news/2023/10/30/fact-sheet-biden-harris-administration-executive-order -directs-dhs-lead-responsible.

| 14 | Ross C. In new order on AI, Biden is scrambling to catch up to emerging risks in health care. *Stat+.* October 30, 2023. Accessed April 3, 2024. https://www .statnews.com/2023/10/30/executive-order-regulating-ai-artificial-intelligence -health-care/#:~:text=In%20new%20order%20on%20AI,emerging%20risks%20 in%20health%20care&text=President%20Biden%20ordered%20the,and%20 other%20health%2Drelated%20businesses.

| 15 | Repici A, Badalamenti M, Maselli R, et al. Efficacy of real-time computer-aided detection of colorectal neoplasia in a randomized trial. *Gastroenterology.* 2020 Aug;159(2):512-520.e7. doi: 10.1053/j.gastro.2020.04.062.

| 16 | Wu E, Wu K, et al. How medical AI devices are evaluated: Limitations and recommendations from an analysis of FDA approvals. *Nat Med.* 2021 Apr;27(4):582-584. doi: 10.1038/s41591-021-01312-x.

| 17 | Wong A, Otles E, et al. External validation of a widely implemented proprietary sepsis prediction model in hospitalized patients. *JAMA Intern Med*. 2021 Aug 1;18:1065-1070. doi: 10.1001/jamainternmed.2021.2626.

| 18 | Shah N, Halamka J, et al. A nationwide network of health AI assurance laboratories. *JAMA*. 2024 Jan 16;331(3):245-249. doi: 10.1001/jama.2023.26930.

| 19 | Cerrato P. *Protecting Patient Information: A Decision-Maker's Guide to Risk, Prevention, and Damage Control*. Syngress/Elsevier; 2016.

| 20 | U.S. Health and Human Services. The Security Rule. Accessed November 5, 2024. https://www.hhs.gov/hipaa/for-professionals/security/index.html# :~:text=The%20HIPAA%20Security%20Rule%20establishes,160%2C%20162 %2C%20and%20164.

CHAPTER 4

Digital solutions are reinventing healthcare

Mayo Clinic Platform (MCP), the division we work for, has a bold vision: to create a healthier world where personalized, predictive, and innovative care is accessible to all. Our mission is to enable new knowledge, new solutions, and new technologies that improve patients' lives. To accomplish our mission, MCP is partnering with providers, pharmaceutical companies, medical device companies, health tech startups, patients, and payers to drive innovation around diagnosis, treatment, and operational improvement. All these efforts rest on an unshakable set of core values, which is represented by the acronym RICH TIES.

Respect. Commit to being respectful—toward each other and toward our patients, partners, and customers.

Integrity. Strive to do what is right, ethical, and honest and expect to be held accountable for what we say and do.

Compassion. Create a supportive, caring, and kind environment where we listen with empathy and act without judgment.

Healing. Aspire to create a healthier world for all, in everything we do.

Teamwork. Believe in the power of working together. Our shared vision and collaboration make us one team.

Innovation. Innovate with purpose with our colleagues and our partners. That purpose serves as our true north.

Excellence. Seek exceptionalism in ourselves, our partners, and our collaborators. Together, we can change the world.

Stewardship. Drive the transformation of healthcare around the world by bringing together local and global communities.

We follow a code of conduct that's consistent with these values, referred to as the Digital Hippocratic Oath. It states:

> As a Mayo Clinic Platform stakeholder, I pledge to maintain the highest standards of professionalism and uphold the principles of autonomy, non-maleficence, beneficence, and justice in my healthcare work. I acknowledge the paramount importance of patient data privacy, confidentiality, and security in our work to enable solutions and technologies that improve patients' lives and alleviate clinician burden. I promise to comply with all ethical and legal standards, including HIPAA. I recognize the needs of the patient as our guiding light and will apply all necessary measures to create a healthier world of personalized, predictive, and innovative care that is accessible to all.
>
> Mayo Clinic Platform is committed to safeguarding the integrity and privacy of data. Mayo Clinic Platform provides data stewardship for patients and our partners, respecting data ownership and intellectual property. I vow to actively mitigate bias and to strive toward creating an equitable healthcare ecosystem that prioritizes patient well-being and the privacy of data.
>
> While I recognize the potential benefits of technology and data, I am also mindful of the potential risks. Therefore, I will strive to reduce these risks by engaging in continuous learning and collaborations that align with Mayo Clinic Platform values.
>
> I acknowledge that my work has a significant impact on patients' lives, and I commit to these principles and our collective shared values: Respect, Integrity, Compassion, Healing, Teamwork, Innovation, Excellence, and Stewardship. I take full responsibility for my actions and will strive to consistently act in accordance with these values. By doing so,

I hope to contribute to the positive transformation of the healthcare industry and find fulfillment in serving as a responsible steward for future generations.

These values and this philosophy have served as the foundation for a long list of digital solutions that are having an impact on the lives of patients globally. Many of these solutions are summarized in Figure 4.1.

ADVANCED CARE AT HOME

Telemedicine has been around for a long time, but it became much more popular when the COVID-19 pandemic started. Telecare accelerated from 3%-4% of visits in January 2020 to 90% in April, to a new normal of 20% in 2021. By one estimate, 43% of adults in the United States used such services in 2022, and that number is likely to grow over time.[1] In 2023, the telemedicine field was valued at about $115 billion.[2] While patients receive most of these services for relatively minor medical problems, individuals with serious needs can also benefit from care provided in the comfort of their own home.

Research has demonstrated that hospital-at-home programs for patients with specific acute medical conditions can reduce complications and reduce the cost of care by 30% or more.[3] One of the most progressive programs to focus on this transition was spearheaded by Johns Hopkins Hospital in 1994. Bruce Leff, MD, and his colleagues tested this program with 455 elderly patients from three Medicare-managed systems and a Veterans Affairs medical center.[4] They found that the home model met quality-of-care standards comparable to those expected of in-hospital programs.

MCP is also involved in the development of a hospital-at-home program, called Advanced Care at Home. It tracks heart rate, blood pressure, pulse oximetry, temperature, and respiratory rate in its patient population, using Bluetooth-enabled devices wirelessly connected to the Mayo/Medically Home system. It also uses tablets, a backup battery system, and a Wi-Fi phone. There are, however, critical differences between many home-care programs and the Mayo Clinic system. Many hospital-at-home programs are targeted and designed for low-acuity hospital patients. They use physician house calls as the clinical delivery model. They have a short patient engagement period (2-4 days).

The Medically Home-affiliated setup is designed to handle an extended length of stay that includes acute, post-acute, and preventative care. It

FIGURE 4.1

AI-driven solutions at Mayo Clinic Platform to improve and transform care

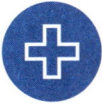

	Advanced Care at Home	In partnership with Medically Home, a model for delivering complex care to patients from the comfort of home has transformed the future of medical care delivery.
	Cardiology AI	In collaboration with partner Anumana, several AI-enabled algorithms that detect heart diseases earlier.
	Early Disease Detection	Using AI-driven technology, these solutions will help identify patients at risk for colorectal cancer, diabetes and opioid use disorder.
	Radiology AI	An AI algorithm to auto-contour head and neck cancers that has been proven superior and more efficient to current software tools and clinical approaches.
	Gastroenterology & Hepatology AI	A digital endoscopy platform that automates image and video acquisition, integrates the data into EHRs so clinicians can access an endoscopy video library.
	Oncology Care	Using deep learning techniques, test results, genetics, and benign breast biopsy findings are harnessed to better identify women at high risk for breast cancer.
	Digital Pathology	Digitized and stored pathology slides from patients to fuel better access for providers, educators, and researchers.

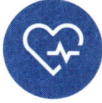

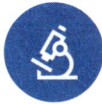

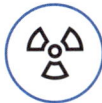

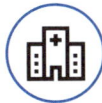

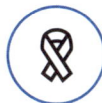

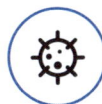

uses a scalable "decentralized" model for high-acuity care and can manage a broad set of diverse use cases and support an extensive patient census. The program uses screening, training, contracting, quality management, and technology and converts "post-acute" community-based supply providers into "acute-level" providers, bringing goods and services to high-acuity patients at home while focusing heavily on the role of paramedics as the centerpiece of its ability to provide "rapid-response" capabilities. In practical terms, that means paramedics and other providers go into the home while being virtually connected with a centralized medical command center staffed by physicians who guide the care for decentralized patients and the decentralized providers who care for them.

Many of the healthcare services patients would receive in a hospital can be provided in the safety and privacy of their own homes. For example, hospital-at-home care may include meals, imaging services, blood draws, physical therapy, wound care, medicine management, and social work services. The program also provides patients with:

- A computer tablet for video visits with the Mayo Clinic care team
- A phone that connects directly to the care team
- A personal emergency response bracelet
- Vital sign monitoring devices
- A router for internet access
- A backup power supply
- Hospital-quality services such as lab tests, mobile ultrasounds and X-rays, and intravenous (IV) therapies

The service is offered at Mayo Clinic in Jacksonville, Florida, and Phoenix, Arizona, and at Mayo Clinic Health System in Eau Claire, Wisconsin. As of December 2024, the program has treated several thousand patients. Studies show that hospital-quality care at home reduced infections and falls, improved outcomes, and increased patient satisfaction while lowering hospital readmission rates.

One of the challenges in choosing a hospital-at-home service is determining who are the best candidates. Advanced Care at Home is a program for people who are sick enough to be in a hospital setting but not so sick that they need surgery, invasive procedures, or advanced imaging. People who enter the program might have an acute-level condition that requires inpatient-quality care. Examples include heart failure, pneumonia, a bloodstream infection, and bronchitis. Among the services offered:

- 24/7 virtual care
- In-person advanced practice provider, nursing, and community paramedic care
- A care plan and schedule designed around each patient's needs
- Pharmacy and medicine management
- Targeted individualized patient education

Additional services, as needed, may include:

- Physical, occupational, and speech therapy
- IV infusion services
- Laboratory testing
- Meals and nutrition
- Mobile imaging and ultrasounds
- Behavioral health
- Social work
- Specialty consultations

The care team is led by Mayo Clinic doctors and includes nurse practitioners, physician assistants, nurses, and other healthcare and service professionals. A patient has access to the team in the Advanced Care at Home command center anytime, day or night. The care may also include in-home visits by a nurse practitioner, a physician assistant, or other healthcare professionals, depending on an individual's needs.

Staff members in the command center direct each episode of care in the home and coordinate with a healthcare professional who is in the home. Each episode of care is detailed in a patient's electronic health record.

Patients may enter the program from the hospital, from the emergency department, or from a doctor's office. Involvement with the program may include three phases.

Acute phase

Depending on the diagnosis, this phase could last up to 6 days. The care team coordinates the appointments in the patient's home to suit their schedule. The first appointment is with a paramedic team, which conducts a home safety assessment to ensure that the patient has a setting suitable for this type of care. This includes a stable internet connection, running water, and sufficient space to limit the risk of falling.

The paramedics also set up equipment they need and coach the individual on how to use it. Examples are a computer tablet on which they will hold video meetings with the care team, a router to provide internet service, various devices for remote monitoring of vital signs, a personal emergency response system (PERS) device for rapid response, and any needed durable medical equipment. After this first visit, the team visits the patient's home each day to address their care needs, which may involve infection control, respiratory therapy, and infusions.

Restorative phase

During the next 25 to 30 days, the patient may be enrolled in remote patient monitoring. Vital signs are remotely monitored through connected devices and the patient has access to the care team by video.

Return to primary care

When a patient is discharged from the Advanced Care at Home program, follow-up care is then provided by their usual primary care team. Additional details about the program, including insurance coverage, are available on the program's website.[5]

ONLINE CARDIOLOGY SERVICES

Ever since William Harvey discovered the essential role of the heart in circulation, clinicians and medical scientists have been seeking new ways to improve the detection and treatment of life-threatening disorders such as heart attacks, heart failure, and related conditions. Like most diseases, these disorders do not appear out of nowhere. Typically, they're preceded by numerous warning signs and symptoms, many of which are too subtle for clinicians to detect without assistance. Over the years, stethoscopes, electrocardiography (ECG) machines, and numerous other devices have improved early detection, but each has its limitations. Machine learning is taking early diagnosis to a new level of sophistication, ushering in what some thought leaders are calling a "golden age" in medicine.

A few years ago, Mayo Clinic developed several artificial intelligence (AI)-enabled algorithms to help diagnose cardiac problems and spun off these services into a company called Anumana.

In a video posted on Anumana's website, Paul Friedman, MD, professor of medicine and chair of the Department of Cardiovascular Medicine at Mayo Clinic, explains that the body is constantly providing physiological clues about cardiovascular status, including heart rate, heart rate variability, electrical signals, and changes in respiration, all of which can be monitored and integrated into an AI-driven algorithm to improve early detection. Mayo Clinic created Anumana to offer its cardiology algorithms to healthcare providers around the world. By tapping data from a very large pool of patients, these algorithms have been able to detect subtle changes in cardiovascular status, which in turn can help detect atrial fibrillation, an abnormal heart rhythm, cardiac amyloidosis (which interferes with normal cardiac functioning by causing deposits of a protein called amyloid), and a weak heart pump (a condition called asymptomatic left ventricular systolic dysfunction, or ALVSD). The researchers and physicians at Mayo Clinic and Anumana are also developing digital tools for early detection of pulmonary hypertension, hypertrophic cardiomyopathy, myocarditis, aortic stenosis, and hyperkalemia, which we discuss in more detail further on in this chapter.

Anumana leverages the largest combined dataset of electrophysiological data, longitudinal patient history, and outcomes in the world. The dataset was developed based on exclusive, multiyear data partnerships with leading academic medical centers and Anumana's parent company, nference. The resulting real-world evidence generation platform, nSights, includes information about 11 million patients spanning 20+ years and transforms unstructured data (i.e., clinical notes, echocardiogram reports) and semistructured (i.e., lab tests, medications, appointments) labeled data. This extensive "deep data" platform fuels Anumana's research and development.

The EAGLE trial, one of the pivotal research studies to demonstrate the value of AI for diagnosing heart disease, showed that detection of ALVSD can be improved by combining AI algorithms with ECG.[6] Asymptomatic ventricular dysfunction only affects 3% of the population and it may not sound serious to a layperson. But people with the disorder may have reduced quality of life and a higher risk of death because their heart's pumping ability is compromised.

In the EAGLE study, Zachi Attia and colleagues at Mayo Clinic used a 12-lead ECG in combination with a type of AI algorithm called a convolutional neural network to identify patients with ALVSD, which they defined as an ejection fraction (EF) at or below 35%. (EF is the percentage of blood that the heart pumps during each beat.) The researchers tested the AI-ECG combination on over 52,000 patients and found measurable benefits.

Anumana is also developing digital tools to improve the diagnosis of hypertrophic cardiomyopathy, a disease in which the heart muscle becomes thickened, or hypertrophied. A thickened heart muscle can make it harder for the heart to pump blood. It's challenging to diagnose because hypertrophy often produces no symptoms. Some patients develop shortness of breath and chest pain, as well as changes in the heart's electrical system, which can lead to a life-threatening irregular heartbeat and sudden death. The chest pain and shortness of breath associated with hypertrophic cardiomyopathy often happen during exercise. It can also cause fainting, especially during or just after exercise or other physical activity, and a sensation of fast, fluttering, or pounding heartbeats called palpitations.

In another study, a combination AI-ECG algorithm from the University of California, San Francisco, and Mayo Clinic used on 216 ECGs was beneficial, suggesting that it can help monitor patients' response to treatment for hypertrophic cardiomyopathy.[7]

EARLY DISEASE DETECTION

Identifying heart disease early is only one tool in the digital tool kit. MCP has also developed algorithms to pinpoint patients at risk for diabetes, lower gastrointestinal (GI) disorders, lung cancer, and stroke. Early recognition of prediabetes and colorectal cancer and polyps is available through Lucem Health, a spinoff from Mayo Clinic. Lucem Health leverages technology from Medial EarlySign, an Israeli company focused on analyzing medical data to identify subtle signs of serious disease.

Prediabetes

By one estimate, about 38% of U.S. adults have prediabetes, and every year, in about 5% of them, it progresses to full-blown diabetes.[8] The Centers for Disease Control and Prevention defines prediabetes as a serious health condition in which blood sugar levels are higher than normal, but not yet high enough to be diagnosed as type 2 diabetes. Patients with prediabetes are at increased risk for diabetes, heart disease, and stroke. Unfortunately, because prediabetes may have no obvious symptoms for years, many people assume there is nothing to worry about. Their philosophy is: If it's not broken, don't fix it. But in reality, your body is already broken if you have the condition, and it is just not talking loud enough for you to notice. Risk factors for prediabetes include being overweight, being 45 or older, having a parent, brother, or sister with type 2 diabetes, being physically active less than 3 times a week, ever having had gestational diabetes (diabetes during pregnancy) or giving birth to a baby who weighed more than 9 pounds, and having polycystic ovary syndrome.

Several blood tests can help identify prediabetes, including a fasting blood sugar test, a glucose tolerance test, and an A1c test. However, many at-risk patients never have these tests. Fortunately, predictive analytics and machine learning tools can help spot people who are most likely to have prediabetes and diabetes. Lucem Health is helping healthcare providers screen their patients for prediabetes.

Colorectal cancer and precancerous polyps

Colorectal cancer is the second leading cause of cancer deaths in the United States, and about 30% of adults are overdue for a standard colorectal cancer screening. Most adults have several options to evaluate their risk of the disease, including the Lucem Health Service, discussed later in the chapter, occult fecal blood testing, Cologuard (a Mayo Clinic-developed test that measures abnormal DNA and blood in the stool), and colonoscopy. Colonoscopy, which is the most sensitive, is recommended for adults age 45 years and older. But too many adults don't want to undergo any of these procedures because they feel healthy and have no GI symptoms. Some people mistakenly believe that they would somehow *know* if they had colorectal cancer, not realizing that many times, the disease starts as tiny "buds" that grow into gigantic trees. Once a cancer is large enough to cause noticeable signs and symptoms, it's often far advanced and may already be life-threatening.

If there ever was a good time to have a colonoscopy, it's now. Digital health experts have developed AI-enabled algorithms to make the procedure even more accurate and more capable of detecting small polyps that gastroenterologists sometimes miss. For a more technical explanation of how these algorithms are benefiting patients, see the TechStop on page 72.

The colorectal cancer screening tool from Lucem Health uses readily available clinical parameters to determine a patient's risk of colorectal cancer.[10,11] ColonFlag was evaluated in a large-scale retrospective study of data from members of Kaiser Permanente Northwest, which included factors such as their age, gender, and complete blood counts. More than

Gastroenterology is one of the specialties that has shown the most promise in terms of application of AI and machine learning. For example, Mayo Clinic's Endoscopy Center is utilizing MCP's resources to explore the value of machine learning in GI care with the assistance of ImaGine, a comprehensive library of endoscopic videos and images linked to clinical data. These data include unedited full-length videos as well as video summaries of the procedure that describe landmarks, specific abnormalities, and anatomical identifiers. Although these projects have tremendous potential for clinicians in routine medical practice and their patients, even more impressive is the work being done in computer-assisted detection (CADe) and computer-aided diagnosis (CADx).

As we've mentioned previously, one of the problems with many of the studies supporting AI-based algorithms is their retrospective design, which is more likely to be flawed because of unanticipated confounding variables. However, in the field of CADe, at least 10 prospective studies have been published, all of which were randomized controlled trials (RCT), the gold standard in clinical research. The preponderance of evidence indicates that CADe is superior to standard colonoscopy, decreasing adenoma miss rates (AMRs) and increasing adenoma detection rates.

Several companies now make software as a medical device (SaMD) systems that enable better detection rates. A SaMD system receives a digital signal from an endoscopy processor and then "outputs a graphical user interface featuring a bounding box at the coordinates of the potential polyp in real time on the existing procedure monitor." In plain English, that means that as the endoscopist is viewing the patient's colon on their computer screen, they also see a visual box surrounding the suspicious lesion, enabling the physician to focus their attention on the specific area (Figure 4.2). The physician can then make a decision about whether the finding is a true or false positive.

Michael Wallace, MD, of Mayo Clinic's Division of Gastroenterology and Hepatology, recently spearheaded a clinical research project that demonstrated the value of AI in colonoscopy. He and his colleagues enrolled 230 patients in an RCT in which half the group had back-to-back colonoscopies, first with AI algorithms used to assist the diagnosis, followed by the procedure without the help of AI. The other group of patients first had the procedure done without AI, followed by the same procedure with the assistance of AI.

The AMR was only 15.5% in the patients who had an AI-assisted colonoscopy, compared with 32.4% when the procedure was initially performed without the benefit of AI. Wallace and colleagues also reported a false-negative rate of 6.8% versus 29.6% in the AI and non-AI groups, respectively. They concluded: "AI resulted in an approximately 2-fold reduction in miss rate of colorectal neoplasia, supporting AI-benefit in reducing perceptual errors for small and subtle lesions at standard colonoscopy."[9]

The AI-based system used in the experiment, GI Genius, relied on a convolutional neural network (CNN) that was previously trained on over 2,600 polyps that were confirmed histologically. In 2021, the Food and Drug Administration approved the CNN to assist clinicians in detecting colon lesions in real time during colonoscopy. The work by Dr. Wallace and others inside and outside Mayo Clinic drives home an important point about AI: It cannot replace an experienced physician's clinical judgment, but studies like this demonstrate that it can have a very real impact when used to augment that judgment.

With the assistance of AI-based algorithms, gastroenterologists who perform colonoscopies are able to detect more precancerous polyps (adenomas), like the ones highlighted in the boxes below.

FIGURE 4.2
AI detection of flat/subtle adenomas

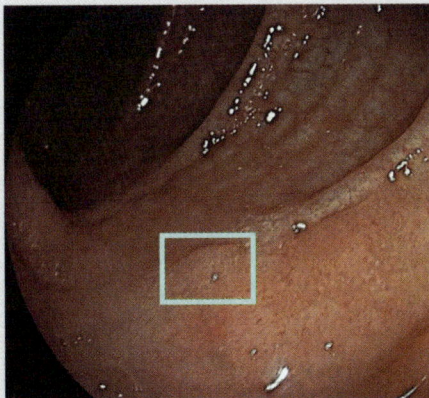

Subtle polyps that might be missed by a gastroenterologist

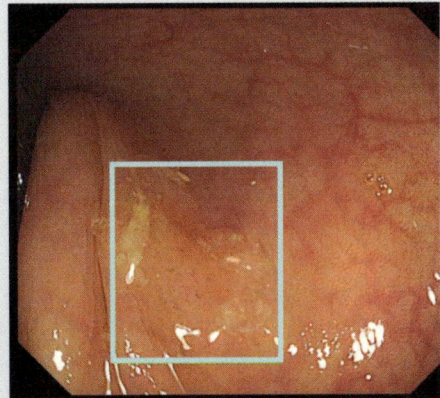

Subtle serrated adenoma of the right colon

17,000 patients were represented in the study, including 900 who already had colorectal cancer. The analysis generated a risk score for patients without the disease to gauge their likelihood of developing it. The researchers compared ColonFlag's ability to predict colorectal cancer with that derived from looking at low hemoglobin (Hgb) levels. (Hgb declines when colorectal cancer causes GI bleeding.) ColonFlag was 34% better than low Hgb at identifying the cancer within a 180-to-360-day period in patients age 50 to 75. The algorithms were more sensitive for detecting tumors in the cecum and ascending colon versus the transverse and sigmoid colon and rectum.

Since that 2017 study, a prospective research project has provided more definitive evidence to support ColonFlag. The ongoing investigation included more than 79,000 patients who had refused colorectal screening. The researchers then applied the ColonFlag algorithms to find individuals who were at high risk of colorectal cancer based on their age, gender, and complete blood counts. Patients who were flagged as high risk were contacted by phone by their physician and asked if they would make an appointment for a screening colonoscopy. The algorithm identified 688 patients who were at highest risk (87th percentile). Of them, 254 consented to have the procedure performed by physicians in the Maccabi Health System; 19 Maccabi patients had cancer (7.5%), and another 15 patients cared for outside the Maccabi system were found to have the cancer through code matching.[12] Goshen and colleagues concluded: "The ColonFlag test is a rapid, efficient and inexpensive test that can be applied to scan electronic medical records to identify individuals at high risk of CRC who would otherwise avoid screening."

TECHNOLOGY TO ENHANCE RADIATION THERAPY

Radiation therapy is one of the most common cancer treatments, used to treat more than half of cancers, yet the labor-intensive expertise in this specialty is in short supply. Digital tools can help address unmet patient needs for the treatment and increase the accuracy of the delivered therapy.

To fully appreciate the impact that AI-enhanced algorithms have on radiation therapy, you first need to understand something about the equipment and technology that deliver radiation to a patient's tumor. Ionizing radiation disrupts cellular DNA, which prevents cancer cells from growing and dividing, which in turn causes solid tumors to shrink. Unfortunately, the same radiation that disrupts tumor growth can also harm nearby healthy tissue, resulting in various complications.

To minimize this risk, computerized programs are used to outline all the anatomical structures closest to the tumor so that an electron beam can more precisely target the tumor and spare the healthy tissues—a procedure called contouring. But there is significant disagreement among providers about how to perform that procedure. Diana Lin and several colleagues in the Department of Radiation Oncology point out that such variation is common and "can affect the resulting plan quality and patient outcomes."[13] Their systematic review found that variations in target volume delineation were responsible for greater treatment toxicity and decreased survival. The medical literature also reveals that major deviations in target delineation occur in up to 13% of radiation therapy plans.

Computer programs are available to help reduce inconsistencies and improve contouring, but these digital tools are far from perfect. Chris Beltran, PhD, chair of the Division of Medical Physics at Mayo Clinic, Florida, points out that the relevant organs and tumors "are critical inputs for the computer models that are currently used to generate radiation dose plans. If organs are not properly identified, the radiation plan may not protect these critical structures or adequately treat the tumor." While computational modeling reduces the risk to healthy tissue, machine learning is now being investigated to make contouring more accurate.

Mayo Clinic and Google Health have developed a joint initiative focusing on research into applying AI to radiation therapy planning. Radiation therapy experts from Mayo Clinic, including radiation oncologists, medical physicists, dosimetrists, and service design experts, are collaborating with Google Health's experts to apply AI to medical imaging. In the first stage of the initiative, Mayo Clinic and Google Health teams are using de-identified data to develop and validate an algorithm to automate the contouring of healthy tissue and organs adjacent to tumors and develop adaptive dosage and treatment plans for patients undergoing radiation therapy for cancers in the head and neck area. The goal of the institutional review board-approved project is to develop an algorithm that will improve the quality of radiation plans and patient outcomes while reducing treatment planning times and improving the efficiency of radiation therapy practice.

The head and neck region was chosen for the Mayo Clinic/Google project because that area of the body contains several sensitive organs that are in close proximity to one another. "Radiation oncologists today painstakingly draw lines around sensitive organs like eyes, salivary glands and the spinal cord to make sure radiation beams avoid these areas. And while this works well, it takes a really long time to get it exactly right," says Cían Hughes, MB, ChB, informatics lead at Google Health.[14] "We see huge potential in using

AI to augment parts of the contouring workflow, and hope that this work will ultimately enable a better patient experience and help patients get the treatment they need sooner."

The potentially revolutionary impact of this new initiative becomes obvious when one considers the fact that virtually all linear accelerators are equipped with an open-source application programing interface (API),* which means it may be possible for hospitals around the world to use the new technology to dramatically improve radiological contouring and make these treatments available to underserved patient populations.

COMPREHENSIVE CANCER CARE AT HOME

Of course, many patients wouldn't need radiation therapy, surgery, or cancer chemotherapy if their cancer or precancerous lesions were detected at a very early stage. As we've pointed out before, early detection is one of the genuine success stories in medicine and has saved countless lives that otherwise would have been lost to late-stage colorectal cancer, cervical cancer, and skin cancer. Unfortunately, early detection protocols still don't exist for several other cancers, including pancreatic cancer. AI-enabled algorithms are beginning to address this problem.

Researchers at the University of Copenhagen, Harvard Medical School, and other institutions have developed an algorithm to help predict the onset of pancreatic cancer. The model suggests that it may be possible to identify patients who will eventually develop the disease at least 3 years before it strikes.[15] Their report states: "These results improve the ability to design realistic surveillance programs for patients at elevated risk, potentially benefiting lifespan and quality of life by early detection of this aggressive cancer."

To create the predictive algorithm, they analyzed clinical data from 6 million Danish patients, including 24,000 with pancreatic cancer, and 3 million patients (3,900 cases) in the United States. Among the risk factors associated with the eventual onset of the disease were jaundice, diabetes, abdominal

---

*Amazon Web Services defines APIs as "mechanisms that enable two software components to communicate with each other using a set of definitions and protocols. For example, the weather bureau's software system contains daily weather data. The weather app on your phone 'talks' to this system via APIs and shows you daily weather updates on your phone." https://aws.amazon.com/what-is/api/.

and pelvic pain, anemia, diseases affecting the bile ducts, acute pancreatitis, and liver disease.

Investigators from MIT and Beth Israel Deaconess Medical Center have also developed a promising AI algorithm that may eventually serve as a routine screening tool for pancreatic cancer.[16] Using a type of AI called a neural network, as well as logistic regression, a more traditional statistics test, they found that their model (Prima) was capable of predicting pancreatic duct adenocarcinoma, the most common form of the disease, 6 to 18 months before diagnosis in patients age 40 years and older.

A few forward-thinking healthcare systems are also developing at-home services to help cancer patients receive treatments that have traditionally been provided in a clinic or hospital setting. In 2022, Memorial Sloan Kettering Cancer Center created a pilot program to administer chemotherapy to patients with neuroendocrine and breast cancers.[17] Similarly, Mayo Clinic is developing a program to shift much of a patient's cancer care to their home. The Cancer Care Beyond Walls (CCBW) Platform will launch inside the MCP with an aim to reduce the cancer burden by creating new care options for patients, improving access and delivering data to support lower costs. CCBW Platform-enabled solutions will support the delivery of care outside traditional settings while maintaining or improving care coordination, the patient experience, and operational efficiencies. This is an opportunity to leverage new technologies to change the way care is delivered. The goal is to support many of the constraints around staffing and capacity that health systems are facing. Initially, the CCBW Platform will focus on patients currently receiving treatment with a plan to expand capabilities across the continuum from risk assessment and early diagnosis to survivorship and supportive care.

With an understanding of the complexity of oncology care, the CCBW system will support a hybrid care model in which outpatients move seamlessly between facility-based care and their homes. This enables the best patient match for the greatest value and impact on clinical outcomes, payment structures, and clinical care team burden. The CCBW Platform has three components: a marketplace to bring together consumers, oncologists, payers, and local providers/vendors to orchestrate care delivery outside the home; a patient population aggregation platform that gathers data and generates insights to support enhanced care delivery and clinical research; and a population risk platform that aims to address population-level outcomes and costs. The goal is to provide end-to-end services and solutions to ensure high-quality care from cancer care providers, education to drive early detection, and proper coverage and reimbursement for services.

Cancer has become a chronic disease. Many patients need active care over a much longer time period, and they want that care to be delivered in a way that supports their quality of life and particular needs. Enabling patient choice with new technologies and driving data to generate insights are key value propositions and top priorities for the CCBW Platform. Getting beyond a traditional exam room or infusion chair to deliver cancer care opens opportunities for flexible, adaptive digital solutions that can deliver staffing optimization, growth capacity, and fewer high-cost care episodes.

AI ENTERS THE PATHOLOGIST'S WORLD

Many people don't feel comfortable thinking about pathology and lab testing. For one thing, it can remind them of the last time a doctor or nurse practitioner recommended testing to rule out some scary disease. Or it may dredge up a memory of a long wait to find out if their mammogram or prostate biopsy was positive for cancer. One reason for those delays is that pathology services are still antiquated. But AI is changing that scenario. Advances in the technology are poised to speed up diagnosis by improving pathologists' ability to identify specific cell structures by more readily spotting "needle-in-the-haystack" abnormalities on a pathology slide, and most importantly, the accuracy of diagnosis.

Mayo Clinic is in the process of scanning all its pathology slides to create one of the largest datasets in the field, which will allow for the creation of pathology-specific AI. Mayo is also embarking on a major initiative to develop a digital pathology platform that can significantly improve the way clinicians provide pathology services to patients. Mayo Clinic Digital Pathology aims to create a connected AI-driven ecosystem, enabling pathologists to tap the potential of intelligent workflows and AI to augment their diagnostic skills with the latest advances in machine learning.

Historically, pathology diagnosis has relied on a pathologist using a microscope to interpret a case by reading glass slides. With digital pathology, the glass slide is scanned, and a digital whole slide image (WSI) is created that can be reviewed from anywhere using a high-fidelity monitor. AI also can be applied to a WSI, allowing it to be analyzed by deep learning algorithms that identify, classify, count, and/or grade target objects, and provide diagnostic interpretation.

As we mentioned earlier in this book, AI can improve the detection of disease by performing in-depth analysis of the millions of pixels in a medical image, something humans are not capable of. In the fields of dermatology, gastro-enterology, and ophthalmology, that has already significantly improved diagnosis. The goal of a digital pathology program is to accomplish the same thing for the many subspecialties of anatomic and clinical pathology.

DIGITAL SOLUTIONS IN THE LARGER HEALTHCARE ECOSYSTEM

Mayo Clinic is certainly not the only healthcare system leading the digital health revolution. LumineticsCore is an algorithm that detects retinopathy, a diabetic eye disease that's the leading cause of blindness in patients with diabetes. Stanford University researchers wanted to find out how effective the digital tool is in motivating patients at risk of retinopathy to follow up with an eye care specialist. They looked at more than 2,200 diabetic patients who were screened with LumineticsCore, formerly IDx-DR, in primary care and endocrinology clinics. Patients who received positive results from the algorithm were about three times as likely to seek the expertise of eye care specialists as patients who didn't have the test performed. That suggests that LumineticsCore really does impact patient decision-making about whether to follow up on their risk of retinopathy.[18]

Further proof of Stanford University's pivotal role in using AI to benefit patients is the Davies Award they recently won for their work in "Thoughtful Application of AI and Telehealth."[19] Presented by the Healthcare Information and Management Systems Society (HIMSS), the award acknowledged the university's work in various arenas, including predicting and preventing clinical deterioration, using AI to help design electronic health records, and transforming emergency department (ED) visits to virtual visits to reduce ED lengths of stay.

Johns Hopkins University has also made a major investment in digital health solutions. In fact, they have an entire department devoted to it, called the Center for Global Digital Health Innovation. As the name suggests, the center places special emphasis on the needs of patients internationally, including in countries with limited resources. The center's Digital Health Exemplars project seeks to identify which factors determine the success of digital health innovations: "Five countries for the study (Brazil, India, Finland, Ghana, Rwanda) have been identified across different geographies, based on the level of digital health maturity and primary healthcare outcomes, and in consultation with several stakeholders including normative agencies and donors, implementors, private sector, and Ministries of Health."[20]

Johns Hopkins is also using AI and data analytics to help identify the risk of suicide among Native Americans: "Longtime tribal-academic research partners will optimize and evaluate NATIVE-RISE, a systems level strategy to suicide prevention that combines service-ready tools based on predictive analytics with risk-stratified evidence-based care for Native American adults."

At the 2023 World Economic Forum in Davos, you might have suspected that the conversation would be about climate change or global conflict. Instead, it was about the impact of AI on our workforce, our economy, and our future. The conclusion: In the short term, the nature of our existing work will change without a major change in workforce, but in the long term, the skills needed to thrive in the workplace will require a different workforce. As Mayo Clinic implements innovative AI-powered solutions—the Digital Pathology Platform, CCBW, and Clinical Trials Beyond Walls—we're seeing a fundamental change in the location of work and the nature of workers. Highly trained subspecialists can serve more patients in more geographies by capturing their knowledge in AI systems and implementing virtual workflows. Just as Amazon created a marketplace where anyone can buy anything anywhere, changing the concept of the retail store, predictive and generative AI will bring the world's experts together with the right patient for the right care at the right time.

This is not about replacing your clinicians with AI. It's about augmenting your clinicians with resources so they can diagnose disease earlier and choose the most effective treatments.

When John Halamka's mother was diagnosed with a brain abscess at a Southern California hospital and the pathology was unclear, they sought the advice of Mayo Clinic by sending glass slides from her brain biopsy to Rochester, Minnesota. The idea behind the Digital Pathology Platform is that any clinician globally can send digitized glass slides to the best expert who can interpret and advise, using AI to rapidly identify abnormalities on the slide.

The combination of nearly infinite computing, curation of data globally, and new workflows that fundamentally change care models is what we mean by "reinventing health care." And along the way, we will ensure that patient privacy is protected, patient preferences are respected, and we will do no digital harm.

KEY TAKEAWAYS

- The Advanced Care at Home program is taking home healthcare to a whole new level, enabling many seriously ill patients who would normally require hospitalization to receive high-quality care in the comfort of their own homes.

- Millions of people have early signs of diabetes but don't know it. Digital tools can now identify the disease earlier, before it gets out of control.

- Algorithms are being used to spot very tiny precancerous polyps in a patient's intestinal tract—minuscule growths that many gastrointestinal (GI) doctors miss.

References

|1| Chang E, Penfold R, Berkman N. Patient characteristics and telemedicine use in the US, 2022. *JAMA Netw Open.* 2024;7(3):e243354. doi: 10.1001/jamanet workopen.2024.3354.

|2| Vaniukov S. Telemedicine market trends and statistics for 2024. Softermii. Accessed May 6, 2024. https://www.softermii.com/blog/telemedicine-trends -and-healthcare-market-statistics.

|3| Cerrato P, Halamka J. *The Digital Reconstruction of Healthcare: Transitioning from Brick and Mortar to Virtual Care.* CRC Press/HIMSS; 2022.

|4| Leff B, Burton L, Mader SL, et al. Hospital at home: Feasibility and outcomes of a program to provide hospital-level care at home for acutely ill older patients. *Ann Intern Med.* 2005 Dec 6;143(11):798-808. doi: 10.7326/0003-4819-143-11 -200512060-00008.

|5| Mayo Clinic Advanced Care at Home. Overview. Accessed May 7, 2024. https:// www.mayoclinic.org/departments-centers/hospital-at-home/sections/overview /ovc-20551797.

|6| Attia ZI, Kapa S, Lopez-Jimenez F, et al. Screening for cardiac contractile dysfunction using an artificial intelligence–enabled electrocardiogram. *Nat Med.* 2019 Jan;25(1):70-74. doi: 10.1038/s41591-018-0240-2.

|7| Siontis K, Abreau S, Attia Z, et al. Patient-level artificial intelligence–enhanced electrocardiography in hypertrophic cardiomyopathy. *JACC Adv.* 2023 Oct 2(8):100582. doi: 10.1016/j.jacadv.2023.100582.

|8| Lucem Health. Use AI to detect prediabetes progression. Accessed May 9, 2024. https://lucemhealth.com/solutions/reveal-prediabetes/.

|9| Wallace M, Sharma P, et al. Impact of artificial intelligence on miss rate of colorectal neoplasia. *Gastroenterology.* 2022 Jul;163(1):295-304.e5. doi: 10.1053/j.gastro.2022.03.007.

|10| Cerrato P, Halamka J. *Reinventing Clinical Decision Support: Data Analytics, Artificial Intelligence, and Diagnostic Reasoning (HIMSS Book Series).* First Edition. Taylor & Francis; 2019.

|11| Hornbrook MC, Goshen R, Choman E, et al. Early colorectal cancer detected by machine learning model using gender, age, and complete blood count data. *Dig Dis Sci.* 2017 Oct;62(10):2719-2727. doi: 10.1007/s10620-017-4722-8.

|12| Goshen R, Choman E, Ran A, et al. Computer-assisted flagging of individuals at high risk of colorectal cancer in a large health maintenance organization using the ColonFlag test. *JCO Clin Cancer Inform.* 2018 Dec;2:1-8. doi: 10.1200/CCI.17.00130.

|13| Lin D, Lapen K, Sherer MV, et al. A systematic review of contouring guidelines in radiation oncology: Analysis of frequency, methodology, and delivery of consensus recommendations. *Int J Radiat Oncol Biol Phys.* 2020 Jul 15;107(4):827-835. doi: 10.1016/j.ijrobp.2020.04.011.

|14| Anastasijevic D. Mayo Clinic, Google launch AI initiative for radiation therapy. Oct 28, 2020. https://newsnetwork.mayoclinic.org/discussion/mayo-clinic-google-launch-ai-initiative-for-radiation-therapy/.

|15| Placido D, Yuan B, et al. A deep learning algorithm to predict risk of pancreatic cancer from disease trajectories. *Nat Med.* 2023 May;29(5):1113-1122. doi: 10.1038/s41591-023-02332-5.

|16| Jia K, Kundrot S, Palchuk MB, et al. A pancreatic cancer risk prediction model (Prism) developed and validated on large-scale US clinical data. *EBioMedicine.* 2023 Dec;98:104888. doi: 10.1016/j.ebiom.2023.104888.

| 17 | Daly B, Huang J, Maiorano J, et al. A treatment-at-home pilot: Barriers to home cancer care. *Oncol Issues*. 2024;39(2):45-53. https://doi.org/10.3928/25731777 -20240422-08.

| 18 | Dow E, Chen K, et al. Artificial intelligence improves patient follow-up in a diabetic retinopathy screening program. *Clin Ophthalmol*. 2023 Nov 2;17:3323- 3330. doi: 10.2147/OPTH.S422153.

| 19 | Health Information and Management Systems Society, Inc. (HIMSS). Stanford Medicine earns Davies award for thoughtful application of AI and telehealth. August 11, 2023. Accessed May 27, 2024. https://www.himss.org/news /stanford-medicine-earns-davies-award-thoughtful-application-ai-and -telehealth.

| 20 | Johns Hopkins Bloomberg School of Public Health. Center for Global Digital Health Innovation. Policies and Practice. Accessed May 29, 2024. https:// publichealth.jhu.edu/center-for-global-digital-health-innovation/policy -practice.

CHAPTER 5

Fixing the misdiagnosis problem

If you've ever had debilitating symptoms and your physician or an advanced practice provider couldn't figure out the cause, you know from firsthand experience how frustrating that can be. And if you've seen numerous clinicians and still haven't received a definitive diagnosis, you're in good company—although clearly, there's nothing good about it.

Millions of patients have been through a similar ordeal. Take 12-year-old Rory Staunton, for example, whose case was described in a textbook. He cut himself playing basketball and later developed abdominal pain, fever, and vomiting.[1] A pediatrician and a physician at the local emergency department who saw Rory ascribed his elevated white blood cell count and other symptoms to a common viral infection and sent him home with instructions to drink fluids and take pain relievers. According to the textbook, "Within days of release from the emergency department, he died from an overwhelming streptococcal infection." Unfortunately, this is only the tip of the iceberg.

A 2015 report from the National Academy of Medicine points out that every year, about 5% of adult outpatients in the United States experience a diagnostic error.[2] The same report found that diagnostic mishaps contribute to about 1 in 10 patient deaths, cause as much as 17% of adverse events seen in hospitalized patients, and affect approximately 12 million adult outpatients a year, which translates into 1 in 20 Americans. About 71,400 of the 850,000 patients who die in U.S. hospitals every year had a significant health condition that went undetected. A more recent study found that about 371,000 people die annually as a result of a misdiagnosis, and 424,000 are permanently disabled.[3] One reason that statistics on diagnostic errors vary so much is that there isn't an agreed-upon way to measure the problem, and without accurate metrics, there's no reliable way to determine if potential solutions are having a significant impact.

HOW TO MEASURE THE MISDIAGNOSIS PROBLEM?

Traditionally, we've relied on several metrics to estimate the incidence of diagnostic mistakes: medical records review, malpractice claims data, insurance claims, autopsies, reviews of diagnostic tests, reviews of medical imaging, clinician surveys, and patient surveys. Each has its strengths and weaknesses, and most are labor intensive.[4]

Medical records

The Harvard Medical Practice Study (1991), which examined more than 30,000 patient records, found that diagnostic errors contributed to 17% of all identified adverse effects, while an analysis of Colorado and Utah hospitals (2000) concluded that diagnostic errors caused 6.9% of adverse reactions.[5] A more recent investigation in the Netherlands found that 6.4% of all adverse effects reported in a hospital setting were related to diagnosis.[5] When the researchers divided these errors into subcategories, they found that about 96% were a result of human failures. The primary causes of diagnostic adverse effects were classified as "knowledge-based failures (physicians did not have sufficient knowledge or applied their knowledge incorrectly) and information transfer failures (physicians did not receive the most current updates about a patient)."[6]

Malpractice claims

An analysis of 25 years of medical malpractice lawsuits gleaned from the National Practitioner Data Bank found that the most common reason for payment of a claim was diagnostic error (28.6%). The same analysis concluded that such errors were far more likely to be linked to patients dying when compared with other issues, including surgery, drugs, and treatment options. The Institute of Medicine report also pointed out that about 70% of diagnostic error malpractice claims happened in an outpatient setting, but "inpatient diagnostic error claims were more likely to be associated with patient death."[2] A Doctors Company review of malpractice claims in 10 medical specialties found that 9% occurred in obstetrics and 61% in pediatrics. The most common disorders represented in malpractice claims included acute myocardial infarction, cancer, appendicitis, and acute stroke.[7]

Health insurance claims

It's now possible to link insurer databases to federal death registries. These types of correlations have been used to detect potential diagnostic errors related to congestive heart failure, 30-day hospital readmissions, and other expensive complications that are now of keen interest to the U.S. government. One such analysis looked at patients admitted to the hospital for stroke who had received previous treatment in the emergency department (ED) and been released 30 days earlier. More than 12% of the admissions may have been the result of a missed diagnosis, and 1.2% reflected "probable missed diagnoses."[8]

Diagnostic testing

Reports about the frequency of laboratory test errors vary widely, but most of these analyses agree that the preanalytic and postanalytic phases of lab testing are the most vulnerable to error. One analysis found that 62% of errors occurred during the preanalytic phase, 15% during actual testing, and 23% during the postanalytic phase.[9] Test follow-up is also an issue that contributes to diagnostic errors, with failure rates as high as 23% among hospital patients and 16.5% in the ED.[10]

Physician surveys

A survey of nearly 600 physicians found that diagnostic errors were most likely to occur in cases of pulmonary embolism, cancer, drug reaction, stroke, and acute coronary syndrome.[10] An independent survey found that more than one-third of physicians had either experienced a diagnostic error themselves or observed one in a family member.[11] It's probably obvious to most readers that surveys are not the most reliable or accurate way to estimate the frequency of diagnostic errors because they're subject to many biases.

Patient surveys

A 1997 survey from the National Patient Safety Foundation found that about 1 in 6 patients (16.6%) reported that they or a close friend or relative had experienced a diagnostic error.[12] In a more recent survey, 23% of respondents said that they or someone close to them had experienced a medical error, about half of which were described as diagnostic mistakes.[13]

Enter AI

Because all these metrics have shortcomings and require considerable resources to implement, there is a growing movement to enlist artificial intelligence-enhanced tools to supplement or even replace them. Ava Liberman at the Department of Neurology at Albert Einstein College of Medicine and David Newman-Toker at Johns Hopkins have developed an AI system that has the potential to replace these legacy approaches to diagnostic error tracking.[14]

Liberman and Newman-Toker's approach uses well-documented symptom/disease pairs that have been shown to occur together during diagnostic mishaps. The Symptom-Disease Pair Analysis of Diagnostic Error, or SPADE, relies on readily available administrative and clinical data from electronic health records (EHRs), billing, and insurance claims to measure the rate at which seemingly benign ED diagnoses are followed up in a short period of time by rehospitalization for a much more serious diagnosis that apparently was missed during the initial patient presentation. For example, dizziness in ED patients sometimes is mistakenly attributed to an inner ear infection when, in fact, its root cause is cerebral ischemia and stroke. As Liberman and Newman-Toker point out: "With untreated TIA [transient ischemic attack] and minor stroke, there is a marked increased short-term risk of major stroke in the subsequent 30 days that tapers off by 90 days. A clinically relevant and statistically significant temporal association between ED discharge for supposedly 'benign' vertigo followed by a stroke diagnosis within 30 days is therefore a biologically plausible marker of diagnostic error. If this missed diagnosis of cerebral ischaemia resulted in a clinically meaningful adverse health outcome (e.g., stroke hospitalisation), this would suggest misdiagnosis-related harm."[14]

For a health system to implement the SPADE approach, it must have access to a large dataset of patient information that includes two specific points in time for each patient: the initial diagnosis and when it was given, and the final diagnosis and its timing. It's also important to have established a "clinically relevant and statistically significant temporal association" between the two events. To establish the symptom/disease pairs worth considering as part of a diagnostic error metric, Liberman and Newman-Toker used look-back and look-ahead analyses; that is, they first studied a specific disease and looked back to determine which symptomatic presentations are most likely to be missed. The look-forward analysis started with a symptom in the patient population to determine which diseases were most likely to be missed. [14] Additional symptoms/disease pairs that are credible candidates for this metrics system include headache/aneurysm, chest pain/myocardial infarction, and fainting/pulmonary embolism.

How large does the dataset need to be in order for this approach to work? At least 5,000 to 50,000 visits, which would generate 50 to 100 diagnostic error outcome events. This estimate is based on previous research that found misdiagnosis harm rates of about 0.2% to 2%.

WHAT'S CAUSING THE MISDIAGNOSIS PROBLEM?

Before we can fix the misdiagnosis dilemma in healthcare, it's important to understand its many causes. In a previous book, [4] we listed several of these issues.

Some patients aren't forthcoming during their medical visits. That can impede both diagnosis and treatment. One of our relatives, for instance, had excessive bleeding after an eye injection to treat macular degeneration. Before the injection, they were asked if they were on any medications or herbal remedies and failed to mention taking ginkgo biloba, which is known to slow down blood clotting. Similarly, another person we know wouldn't admit that he had benign prostatic hyperplasia (an enlarged prostate). But the condition made it impossible to insert a Foley catheter into his bladder as he was being prepared for surgery. The procedure had to be canceled, inconveniencing him and his healthcare team.

Solving this type of problem isn't always simple. Even when physicians encourage their patients to be open, they may still be reluctant to disclose information, for a variety of reasons. Chief among them may be embarrassment about admitting to certain activities that they think the doctor will frown upon, like smoking, having unprotected sex, or heavy drinking. One survey found that "38 percent of patients lied or 'stretched the truth' about following their doctor's orders, while 32 percent lied about their diet or how much they exercised. Another 22 percent lied about smoking, 17 percent lied about sex, 16 percent lied about their intake of alcohol, and 12 percent lied about recreational drug use."[15]

It's also possible that a patient may hold back vital information because they fear the doctor will share the information with a third party such as a law enforcement or insurance company. Many of the concerns about disclosure can be resolved if a patient and doctor develop a strong *trusting* relationship. Unfortunately, this isn't the case for many patients who have yet to find a primary care provider. The take-home message here is clear: If at all possible, find a primary care physician or advanced practice provider and be completely open with them. Odds are, it will improve the likelihood that you'll get an accurate diagnosis.

Of course, healthcare providers can also contribute to the misdiagnosis dilemma by ignoring patient input about signs and symptoms. Or they may have limited knowledge about the disease that a patient has, which is an especially common problem if it's rare or the clinician has had little experience caring for patients who have it. Other possible reasons for a misdiagnosis:

- Incorrect interpretation of medical information because of a clinician's cognitive errors and biases
- Failure to integrate collected medical information into a plausible diagnostic hypothesis
- Not properly communicating the diagnosis to patients
- Lab testing errors
- Communication problems between testing facilities and clinicians
- Poorly designed clinical documentation systems, including EHRs
- Inadequate interoperability between providers
- Failure to integrate the diagnostic process into clinicians' normal workflow
- Poor handoff procedures
- Inadequate teamwork
- Fear on the part of a clinician's subordinates about speaking up when they perceive a diagnostic misstep
- Disruptive physical environment, including noise, bad lighting, distractions
- Poorly located equipment

Cognitive errors contribute significantly to the misdiagnosis problem. Common cognitive errors include anchoring, affective bias, availability bias, premature closure, and confirmation error. During anchoring, a diagnostician will get fixated on initial findings and stay anchored to this line of reasoning even when contrary evidence suggests it's best to change direction. The culture of modern medicine fosters this mindset because it encourages physician overconfidence in their own skill set, and because physicians, like many other leaders, believe the appearance of certainty is the best course of action.

Clinicians, like the rest of society, also can be swayed by their positive and negative emotional reactions to patients, or so-called affective bias. Availability bias is common among clinicians who see the same disorder over and over within a short time frame or who have done research on a specific disorder. Premature closure occurs when a practitioner is too quick to accept the first plausible explanation for all the presenting signs and symptoms. Confirmation error "is the tendency to look for confirming evidence to support a theory rather than disconfirming evidence to refute it, even if the latter is clearly present."[16]

To help fix these thinking errors, one needs to understand the way clinicians—and the rest of us—think. Cognition can be divided broadly into two systems: fast thinking and slow thinking, also referred to as Types 1 and 2. With regard to Type 1 thinking, Pat Croskerry, MD, PhD, Department of Emergency Medicine professor at Dalhousie University in Halifax, Nova Scotia, points out: "The system is fast, frugal, requires little effort, and frequently gets the right answer. But occasionally it fails, sometimes catastrophically. Predictably, it misses the patient who presents atypically, or when the pattern is mistaken for something else."[17] The shortcomings of intuitive thinking were dramatically illustrated in an analysis of over 20,000 patients with acute coronary syndromes. Investigators found that 1,763 did not present with the usual chest pain; in this subgroup, nearly 1 in 4 were not identified as having experienced an acute coronary event (23.4%).[18]

Type 2 reasoning is particularly effective in scenarios in which the patient's presentation follows no obvious disease script, the pattern is atypical, and there's no unique pathognomonic signpost to clinch the diagnosis. It usually starts with a hypothesis that is then subjected to analysis with the help of critical thinking, logic, multiple branching, and evidence-based decision trees and rules. This analytic approach also requires an introspective mindset that is sometimes referred to as metacognition, namely, the "ability to step back and reflect on what is going on in a clinical situation."[17]

This skill set also lets clinicians run through a list of common cognitive errors that can easily send them in the wrong direction. But because Type 2 reasoning is a much slower process, it's often a challenge to implement, especially in high-stress, high-volume settings. For the slow, reflective, Type 2 mode to be most effective, it requires a well-rested clinician who isn't distracted, doesn't have an unreasonably heavy workload, and has had enough sleep to fully use their analytical skills and memory. Too few work environments satisfy these prerequisites.

Another reason for misdiagnosis errors is lack of training in clinical reasoning for medical school and allied healthcare students. One survey from five European countries found many barriers that interfere with the creation of a formal curriculum that covers clinical reasoning, including lack of time, "difficulties in organizing clinical reasoning teaching and assessment due to lack of physical space, adequate hardware/software infrastructure, and workflows," and resistance from decision-makers within the university or national healthcare systems who don't want to change.[19] That's the case because many veteran clinicians believe it's enough for students to learn informally through mentoring from more experienced diagnosticians. Other studies have found that only 1 in 4 medical schools have courses that "explicitly teach clinical reasoning."[19]

In 2015, the National Academy of Medicine issued a detailed report, *Improving Diagnosis in Health Care,* in which it highlighted the need to "enhance healthcare professional education and training in the diagnostic process." Similarly, it addressed the resistance to such educational efforts by stating the need to "establish a work system and culture that supports the diagnostic process and improvements in diagnostic performance."[2]

On a more positive note, organizations like the Society to Improve Diagnosis in Medicine (SIDM) have developed a wide variety of tools to address this very problem. For example, *Root Cause Analysis of Cases Involving Diagnosis: A Handbook for Healthcare Organizations,* published by SIDM, provides practical instructions on how to find cases of diagnostic errors—and successes. It pinpoints the mistakes along the diagnostic process that triggered the errors and explains how to evaluate the "cognitive aspects of the decision that were made, both the subconscious, intuitive aspects of clinical reasoning as well as the deliberate conscious counterparts." The handbook also offers guidelines for how to intervene.[20]

DIAGNOSING PATIENTS IS HARD WORK

One thing we don't want to overlook, after reviewing all the troublesome statistics on misdiagnosis and all the discussion about medical professionals needing more training on diagnosis, is the fact that often, diagnosing a patient's condition can be very difficult for even the most conscientious, well-informed clinician. Medicine is as much an art as it is a science. And the reality is that some clinicians are better artists than others.

That said, what can patients do to improve their odds of getting an accurate diagnosis? SIDM provides practical advice on the subject:

> One way to protect patients and families from experiencing diagnostic errors is to educate them about the risks and provide them with tools and resources to push for more answers when they feel like something "isn't right." In the hospital setting, a critical partner in pushing for diagnostic safety are Patient and Family Advisory Councils or PFACs. Because PFACs are composed of people with lived experience of illness or disease, they bring first-hand knowledge of what it is like to go through the diagnostic process. While PFACs provide input and guidance to hospitals on a host of topics, they can be key advocates for improving diagnostic safety through a variety of activities and efforts.[20]

Another option is for patients to enlist a patient advocate to get involved in meetings designed to find the root cause of a misdiagnosis. "Experienced advocates will be familiar with medical language, standard medical care processes, and safety analyses, and can report back to (or explain things to) the patient or family as needed."[20]

Diagnostic errors will always be with us, the result of a complex set of clinical, social, and cultural issues. But the solutions outlined here can help mitigate the problem, likely saving lives in the process.

KEY TAKEAWAYS

- Millions of people are misdiagnosed every year. Encouraging patients to push back when they sense something isn't right is helping to solve this national epidemic.

- In a hospital setting, Patient and Family Advisory Councils (PFACs) are being set up to encourage more accurate diagnoses.

- Because PFACs are composed of people with lived experience of illness or disease, they bring firsthand knowledge of what it's like to go through the diagnostic process.

References

|1| Trowbridge R, ed. *Teaching Clinical Reasoning*. American College of Physicians; 2015.

|2| Committee on Diagnostic Error in Health Care; Board on Health Care Sciences; Institute of Medicine; National Academies of Sciences, Engineering, and Medicine. Balogh EP, Miller BT, Ball JR, eds. *Improving Diagnosis in Health Care*. National Academies Press; 2015.

|3| Merelli A. Misdiagnoses cost the U.S. 800,000 deaths and serious disabilities every year, study finds. *Stat News*. July 21, 2023. Accessed June 27, 2024. https://www.statnews.com/2023/07/21/misdiagnoses-cost-the-u-s-800000-deaths-and-serious-disabilities-annually-study/.

|4| Cerrato P, Halamka J. *Reinventing Clinical Decision Support: Data Analytics, Artificial Intelligence, and Diagnostic Reasoning (HIMSS Book Series)*. First Edition. Taylor & Francis; 2019.

|5| Leape LL, Brennan TA, et al. The nature of adverse events in hospitalized patients: Results of the Harvard Medical Practice Study II. *New England Journal of Medicine*. 1991;324(6):377-384.

|6| Zwaan L, de Bruijne M, Wagner C, et al. Patient record review of the incidence, consequences, and causes of diagnostic adverse events. *Arch Intern Med*. 2010;170(12):1015-1021. doi: 10.1001/archinternmed.2010.146.

|7| Troxel D. Input submitted to the Committee on Diagnostic Error in Health Care from the Doctors Company Foundation. 2014, April 28.

|8| Newman-Toker DE, Moy E, Valente E, et al. Missed diagnosis of stroke in the emergency department: A cross-sectional analysis of a large population-based sample. *Diagnosis*. 2014;1(2):155-166.

|9| Carraro P, Plebani M. Errors in a stat laboratory: Types and frequencies 10 years later. *Clinical Chemistry.* 2007;53(7):1338-1342.

|10| Callen J, Georgiou A, Li J, Westbrook JI. The safety implications of missed test results for hospitalized patients: A systematic review. *BMJ Quality & Safety.* 2011;20(2):194-199.

|11| Blendon R J, DesRoches CM, et al. Views of practicing physicians and the public on medical errors. *New England Journal of Medicine.* 2002;347(24):1933-1940.

|12| Golodner L. How the public perceives patient safety. *Newsletter of the National Patient Safety Foundation.* 1997;1(1):1-4.

|13| Betsy Lehman Center for Patient Safety and Medical Error Reduction. The Public's Views on Medical Error in Massachusetts. Cambridge (MA): Harvard School of Public Health. 2014.

|14| Liberman AL, Newman-Toker DE. Symptoms-Disease Pair Analysis of Diagnostic Error (SPADE): A conceptual framework and methodological approach for unearthing misdiagnosis-related harms using big data. *BMJ Quality & Safety,* 2018; Jul;27(7):557-566. doi: 10.1136/bmjqs-2017-007032.

|15| Schwartz SK. When patients lie to you. Roswell Park Comprehensive Cancer Center. 2010. Accessed July 2, 2024. https://www.roswellpark.org/partners -in-practice/white-papers/when-patients-lie-you.

|16| Wachter RM, Gupta K. *Understanding Patient Safety.* 3rd ed. McGraw-Hill Education; 2018.

|17| Croskerry P. A universal model of diagnostic reasoning. *Acad Med.* 2009 Aug;84:1022-1028. doi: 10.1097/ACM.0b013e3181ace703.

|18| Brieger D, Eagle KA, Goodman SG, et al. Acute coronary syndromes without chest pain, an underdiagnosed and undertreated high-risk group: Insights from the Global Registry of Acute Coronary Events. *Chest.* 2004;126:461-469.

|19| Sudacka M, Adler M, Durning SJ, et al. Why is it so difficult to implement a longitudinal clinical reasoning curriculum? A multicenter interview study on the barriers perceived by European health professions educators. *BMC Med Educ.* 2021 Nov 12;21:575.

| 20 | Graber ML, Castro G. *Root Cause Analysis of Cases Involving Diagnosis: A Handbook for Healthcare Organizations.* Leapfrog Group; 2024. Accessed July 10, 2024. https://www.leapfroggroup.org/sites/default/files/Files/Root%20 Cause%20Analysis%20of%20Cases%20Involving%20Diagnosis%20A%20 Handbook%20for%20Healthcare%20Organizations.pdf.

CHAPTER 6

Personalized medicine and the genomics revolution

"Medicine may be on the cusp of an era of astonishing innovation—the limits of which aren't even clear yet." This quote from the *New York Times* will no doubt be met with skepticism from some patients and medical professionals who have seen too many "revolutions" turn out to be empty promises.[1] But if you take a closer look at the evidence behind the statement, you'll see it's not hype. It's an emerging reality assisted by a variety of digital tools.

A very brief history lesson will help put this enthusiasm into perspective. In 2003, the Human Genome Project was completed. It was the first time the complete genetic blueprint of a human was available. In 2015, the Precision Medicine Initiative was launched to investigate whether all the new genomic data, combined with several lifestyle and environmental factors, might contribute to a person's health and their risk of various diseases. Why is such a program needed? Because until recently, health-care providers have taken a one-size-fits-all approach to patient care, working on the assumption that we're all pretty much the same in terms of our anatomy, bodily functions, and body chemistry. That assumption has been proven wrong.

One-size-fits-all medicine, also called population-based medicine, typically uses a treatment plan that has proven successful for *most* patients. In other words, it assumes that the treatment that works for the average patient will work for every patient. But as many unsatisfied patients will testify, millions of us aren't average and don't respond well to standard treatments. The shortcomings of the one-size-fits-all approach to patient care are well illustrated by the fact that so many patients fail to respond to state-of-the-art therapy for a variety of disorders. By one estimate, the 10 bestselling medications in the United States benefit between 4% and 25% of the patients using them. The current role of statins in the prevention and treatment of heart disease highlights the limitations of population-based medicine. Estimates indicate that only 5% of patients given rosuvastatin (Crestor) will benefit from it.[2] Similarly, just over 4% of patients who take esomeprazole (Nexium) and approximately 11% of those who take duloxetine (Cymbalta) are likely to benefit from these drugs.

What's needed, then, is an approach to patient care that identifies people who will actually benefit from the thousands of drugs, surgical procedures, and lifestyle modifications recommended by clinicians worldwide.[3] That's the lofty goal of precision medicine, and to accomplish it, we'll need to take a holistic, personalized view. In many cases, that will involve studying massive numbers of people to detect significant associations between genetic and environmental risk factors and disease and to detect root causes. If root causes can't be found, we'll need to figure out which individuals will and won't respond well to available management protocols. The Precision Medicine Initiative (now called the All of Us Project) has been collecting data like those we've just described for almost a decade and is making its findings available to researchers, in hopes that the information will eventually have practical applications in patient care.

PUTTING PRECISION MEDICINE TO WORK IN DIABETES CARE

Other investigators also are beginning to figure out how to use all the data on genetics and lifestyle factors in patient care. For instance, research conducted by Jeremy Sussman and his colleagues at the University of Michigan and Tufts Medical Center is pointing us in the right direction. They're using predictive analytics to help identify people at risk of type 2 diabetes (T2D) and to figure out which of them might go on to develop the disease.[4]

Sussman and colleagues analyzed the results of the Diabetes Prevention Program (DPP), a large-scale randomized clinical trial in which over 3,000 patients were given various preventive regimens to determine if it was possible to reduce the incidence of T2D in at-risk patients. The participants were divided into three groups:

1. Group 1 (controls) received standard lifestyle recommendations plus twice-daily placebo pills.

2. Group 2 followed an intensive lifestyle modification program, which included lessons from a case manager on implementing the regimen.

3. Group 3 followed standard lifestyle recommendations and took 850 mg of metformin (an effective oral anti-diabetes drug) twice daily.

All the patients enrolled in the DPP were clearly at risk for T2D. They had a body mass index (BMI) of 24 or higher, a fasting plasma glucose of 96-125 mg/dL, which is considered impaired fasting glucose, and a glucose tolerance test result of 140-199 mg/dL. The test results mean that their bodies didn't tolerate glucose (sugar) well. With readings like these, it's likely that many of the patients would progress to full-blown diabetes.

After nearly 3 years, the estimated cumulative incidence of diabetes was 14.4% in the patients in Group 2 who adhered to the intensive lifestyle program, 21.6% among the patients in Group 3, and 28.9% among the patients in Group 1. Put another way, lifestyle modification reduced the incidence of diabetes by 58% and metformin reduced it by 31%.[5] The problem with these results is that it wasn't possible to separate responders from nonresponders; in other words, the data couldn't be readily personalized. To resolve that issue, Sussman and colleagues designed a diabetes risk model. They started their analysis with several potential risk factors for diabetes that previous research had shown could predict the disease, including:

- Fasting blood glucose levels
- Hemoglobin A1c levels
- Age
- BMI*

---

*Body mass index is a person's weight measured in pounds (or kilograms) divided by their height in inches (or meters) squared. Although there are exceptions, readings of 25 or above are considered overweight and readings of 30 or above indicate obesity.

- Waist-to-hip ratio
- Waist circumference
- Height, sex, race
- Family history of elevated blood glucose
- Smoking status
- Triglyceride levels
- High-density lipoprotein cholesterol levels
- Systolic blood pressure

To determine which patients got the most and least benefit from metformin and lifestyle modification, the researchers divided the group based on their risk before they enrolled in the study, using the risk factors we've just listed to predict their outcomes. Seven of the predictive risk factors had the most impact on risk: fasting blood glucose, hemoglobin A1c, family history of elevated blood glucose, triglyceride levels, height, waist measurement in centimeters, and waist-to-hip ratio. More importantly, the researchers found "that average reported benefit for metformin was distributed very unevenly across the study population, with the quarter of patients at the highest risk for developing diabetes receiving a dramatic benefit (21.5% absolute reduction in diabetes over three years of treatment) but the remainder of the study population receiving modest or no benefit."[4] By way of contrast, the difference in benefit from the intensive lifestyle training between higher- and lower-risk patients was minimal. The diabetes risk prediction tool developed by Sussman and colleagues may eventually help clinicians personalize care of at-risk patients by identifying the ones most likely to benefit from drug therapy and sparing the rest from the negative effects of metformin, which can include abdominal or stomach discomfort, cough or hoarseness, decreased appetite, diarrhea, fast or shallow breathing, and fever or chills.

In their *New England Journal of Medicine* report documenting the results of the DPP, William Knowler and associates said: "An estimated 10 million persons in the United States resemble the participants in the Diabetes Prevention Program in terms of age, body-mass index, and glucose concentrations, according to data from the third National Health and Nutrition Examination Survey. If the study's interventions were implemented among these people, there would be a substantial reduction in the incidence of diabetes."[5] The data from the DPP strongly suggest that the population approach to diabetes prevention they studied would subject millions of patients to unnecessary and potentially harmful drug therapy. On the flip side, applying a predictive analytics model that includes the seven risk factors we've previously mentioned would enable clinicians to target the patients most likely to benefit.

Management of heart disease is also entering the era of precision medicine. The seeds of that model were sown in 1948, when the Framingham Heart Study began collecting data on heart disease risk factors. Since then, its authors have tracked the health of over 5,000 adults through physical examinations, lab tests, and lifestyle interviews. In 1971, the study enrolled another 5,000-plus participants: the adult children of the original participants. In 2002, a third generation was added to the cohort. This landmark research has identified several risk factors that contribute to heart disease, including hypertension (high blood pressure), hypercholesterolemia (high cholesterol), obesity, diabetes, physical inactivity, and smoking. (Keep in mind that critics have questioned whether the Framingham Study was representative of the U.S. population.) In 2025, that may sound unimpressive, because most Americans recognize there are health risks associated with being sedentary and using tobacco. But detecting a relationship between these root causes and heart disease was nothing short of transformational in its day. It's easy to forget that there was a time in the not-too-distant past when popular magazines ran ads with headlines like "More Doctors Smoke Camels Than Any Other Cigarette" and images of Santa Claus promoting a popular brand of cigarettes.

Applying the Framingham Heart Study findings to patient care has resulted in dramatic reductions in the death and disease burden for heart disease in recent decades. But it's time for this holistic approach to take a leap into the 21st century with the addition of risk factors based on genetic and genomic data. Recent research on hypertrophic cardiomyopathy (HCM) is a good example of this new direction.

During HCM, the myocardium (heart muscle) gets thick or hypertrophic. That makes it difficult for the heart to pump blood. Signs and symptoms of HCM include shortness of breath, chest pain, fainting, and sudden cardiac death. Although the disease can have many causes, familial HCM is inherited as an autosomal dominant trait. If you're the child of someone with HCM, you have a 50% chance of inheriting the trait and getting the disease. One of the genes involved in HCM encodes for sarcomere proteins, which are part of the tissue in the heart, and if the gene is mutated, the heart muscle will be damaged.

In an effort to customize treatment for patients with symptomatic obstructive HCM, MyoKardia (a subsidiary of Bristol Myers Squibb) developed a unique compound that targets one underlying cause of the disease: abnormal sarcomere contractibility (abnormal contractions in the heart muscle). In animal studies, the new compound, MYK-461, inhibited that process and suppressed HCM. Human studies led to the approval of the drug by the Food and Drug Administration (FDA) to treat obstructive HCM. The drug is sold under the generic name mavacamten and brand name Camzyos.

UNDERSTANDING THE INTERLOCKING CAUSES OF DISEASE

Heart disease is one of the most complex disorders to manage because there are so many interlocking risk factors and contributing causes, and they vary from person to person. Understanding how much each of the factors contributes to a particular individual's risk is crucial in order to optimize care. Consider two patients: Mary Mendez and John Bonomo. Both have heart disease, and their symptoms are similar, but the reasons for their conditions are different. Mary has a genetic mutation that's 70% responsible for her disease and its symptoms, her diet rich in saturated fat and sedentary lifestyle each contribute 5% risk, and Mary's severe chronic stress contributes 20%. In John's case, his inability to cope with physical and psychosocial stress contributes 45%, 35% of the risk is from his poor diet, and 20% is from a combination of genetic mutations called single nucleotide polymorphisms (SNPs). Clearly, Mary and John need different approaches to disease prevention and treatment.

Mary and John aren't real patients, but their profiles aren't completely hypothetical. Familial hypercholesterolemia (FH) is a genetic autosomal dominant disorder that affects 1 in 200-300 people in its milder form. It causes severely elevated plasma levels of low-density lipoprotein (LDL) cholesterol—typically 300-400 mg/dL—and premature heart disease. If Mary has FH, the most important contributor to her heart disease is a genetic mutation that disrupts the production of the LDL receptor on the surface of her cells. For someone like her, a diet low in saturated fat will be of only minimal benefit. To be effective, a treatment would need to target Mary's genetic mutation and its effects on her body (her heart disease). That's where a relatively new family of drugs, called proprotein convertase subtilisin/kexin type 9 (PCSK9) inhibitors, comes in.

PCSK9 is a protein that helps regulate plasma LDL levels. It seems to control the number of LDL receptors on cell surfaces. The more receptors on the surface of liver cells, the faster the liver can remove LDL cholesterol from the bloodstream and the lower a person's risk of heart disease-promoting high cholesterol. In patients like Mary who have a mutation in the gene responsible for production of PCSK9, the result is overexpression of PCSK9, which increases their LDL cholesterol levels. PCSK9 inhibitors are a precise way to treat that problem.

Physical and psychosocial stress also can contribute to heart disease, as is the case with our patient John. By one estimate, psychosocial stress is responsible for 30% of the proportion of heart attacks within a population that can be attributed to this risk factor.[6] But individual reactions to stress and the ability to cope with it are highly variable. Some people's bodies produce a lot of the hormone cortisol in response to stress, whereas other people's bodies do not.

In an average person, cortisol follows a pattern of diurnal cycling, that is, blood levels of the hormone increase when they wake up and gradually drop throughout the day. But in approximately 17% of the population, that's not the case.[7] If John is a "stress responder," meaning that his body produces a lot of cortisol when triggered, then a stress management program and cognitive behavior therapy may reduce his heart disease signs and symptoms. If he hadn't yet developed the disease, these approaches might have helped prevent it.

An individualized approach also may be needed if John's heart disease was triggered, in part, by underlying hypertension. Doctors often prescribe a low-sodium diet to lower blood pressure, but only 11.8% of patients with hypertension are salt-sensitive. Similarly, only 25% of all Americans are salt-sensitive.[8,9] So, it would make sense to test John for sodium sensitivity. If the results are positive, a salt-restricted diet would be justified, but if it has no impact on John's blood pressure, there's no reason to change his diet.

Unfortunately, most physicians and advanced practice providers in routine clinical practice don't have the tools to make the decisions required to personalize treatment for patients like Mary and John. FH usually isn't tested for in primary care practice, blood cortisol levels are rarely measured, there's no readily available test for sodium sensitivity, and genetic testing to detect PCSK9 mutations isn't commonly available or paid for by third-party medical insurers.

THE BIOLOGICAL BASIS FOR PRECISION MEDICINE

The precision/personalized medicine model has a sound biological basis even though its practical applications have yet to be fully realized in many specialties. At the most fundamental level, the population medicine model is functional but flawed. All humans have basic biochemical, metabolic, and genetic commonalities. They're what allows clinicians to treat most patients as though they were the "average" patient. Yet variations among individuals are significant and they're rarely taken into account when approaches to prevention and therapy are developed.

One of the reasons a one-size-fits-all approach to patient care is inadequate is that we're not all one size. Read a human anatomy textbook and you may get the impression that healthy people of the same weight and height have stomachs, livers, and hearts that are the same size and shape. But opening up actual human bodies shows otherwise. Similarly, a clinical chemistry reference chart suggests that all healthy adults have a serum calcium level between 8.6 and 10.0 mg/dL, for example, though by definition, that range is only a statistical convention that includes 97.5% of the population tested. The other 2.5% of healthy people will have readings outside that range. In a U.S. population of 319 million, that means nearly 8 million Americans have blood chemistry levels outside the normal range but they're still healthy.

Clinical chemistry values also are based on a numerical sample of healthy people, but if the sample is too small, it may not represent the range of the entire U.S. population. If serum calcium levels are between 8.6 and 10.0 mg/dL among 1,000 healthy adults, what would the range be among 800,000 sampled adults? We don't really know, yet clinicians continue to base diagnostic and treatment decisions on the assumption that relatively small sample sizes are representative of the entire population.

The "normal" blood levels of several nutrients have been questioned for the same reason. For instance, two early studies that were used to set the recommended dietary allowance for vitamin A involved 16 and 8 volunteers, respectively, which is hardly a representative sample of the human population.

Genetic individuality is at the heart of much of the biochemical, anatomical, physiological, and metabolic individuality observed among humans. Exposure to various environmental factors and their interaction with a person's genes is likely responsible for the rest. The most extreme examples of biochemical and metabolic individuality brought on by genetic variants are inborn errors of metabolism. Phenylketonuria (PKU), for instance, results from a genetic mutation that codes for the enzyme phenylalanine hydroxylase. Without this enzyme, which is needed to convert the amino acid

Inherited traits and genetically induced risk factors are carried on genes located on chromosomes. Each gene is a strand of DNA, composed of deoxyribose, a phosphate group (which consists of phosphorus and oxygen), and nucleotides.

The four bases in DNA are adenine (A), thymine (T), guanine (G), and cytosine (C). They're paired off in a regular pattern, with A and T always bonded together and G and C bonded together. Each strand of DNA contains numerous pairings of A/T and C/G. These bases and their sequence in the DNA molecule act as a code that determines which proteins a cell will synthesize. During the process of transcription, a DNA strand becomes unzipped; that is, it divides down the middle and is copied into RNA.

RNA is decoded by ribosomes in the cell's cytoplasm, the space outside the nucleus, and translated into amino acids, which are linked together to form proteins. Proteins are used by the body to carry out a wide variety of cell functions. Synthesis of each amino acid is determined by specific sequences of nucleotides. For example, the amino acid methionine is created when the nucleotides A, T, and G line up during the translation process.

Unfortunately, a variety of errors can occur during this process. One type of mutation, a single nucleotide polymorphism, occurs when one base is replaced by another. A change in the three-letter genetic code required to produce a specific amino acid can result in that amino acid no longer being manufactured. For instance, if the G (guanine) in the ATG code that translates into the amino acid methionine is replaced with a C (cytosine), the amino acid isoleucine would be made instead.

Replacing one amino acid with another amino acid can seriously disrupt the functioning of a protein or disable it altogether. In sickle cell anemia, for instance, GAG mutates to GTG, which in turn causes a replacement of the amino acid glutamic acid with valine. That single substitution changes the structure and function of the hemoglobin molecule, diminishing its ability to carry oxygen to tissues.

Image courtesy National Human Genome Research Institute. *genome.gov*

FIGURE 6.1
DNA — deoxyribonucleic acid

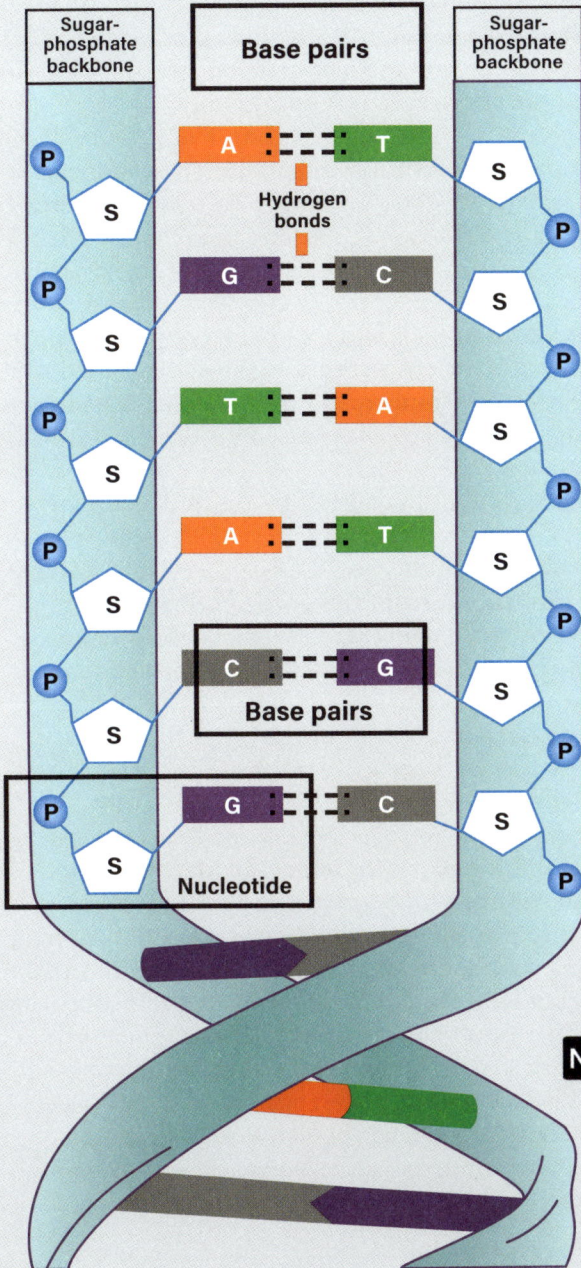

Sugar-phosphate backbone

Base pairs

Sugar-phosphate backbone

A — T

Hydrogen bonds

G — C

T — A

A — T

C — G

Base pairs

G — C

Nucleotide

P S

NIH National Human Genom Research Institute

phenylalanine into tyrosine, a person develops PKU. That, in turn, causes severe intellectual disability. But 100 years ago, Archibald E. Garrod, considered by some as the "father" of precision medicine, pointed out that inborn errors of metabolism are "merely extreme examples of variations of chemical behavior which are probably everywhere present in minor degrees and that this chemical individuality [confers] predisposition to and immunities from the various mishaps which are spoken of as diseases."[10] Put another way, inborn errors of metabolism exist on a continuum, and the rest of humankind is somewhere on that continuum.

Researchers who have studied metabolic individuality point out that any individual human genome probably deviates from a reference genome by about 3 million variants.[11] Many of those variants are the results of genetic variants called SNPs, which are explained in Figure 6.1. Many SNPs have been associated with an increased risk of heart disease, diabetes, kidney disease, high triglyceride levels, and high blood pressure. More specifically, 13 SNPs have been used as part of a risk score, which was able to identify people with an approximately 70% higher risk of having an initial heart disease event.

To illustrate how this genetic/biochemical/metabolic continuum affects individuals, consider some examples:

- SNPs have been identified that disrupt the normal utilization of the B vitamin folic acid. Women who carry this mutation are more likely to miscarry if they have two copies of the defective genetic variant.

- The SNP Ala222Va, which affects the gene responsible for synthesis of the enzyme methylene tetrahydrofolate reductase, not only increases the risk of neural tube defects (NTDs) and heart disease but also reduces the risk of colon cancer. Individuals with the genetic variant may be at lower risk for NTDs and heart disease if they increase their intake of folic acid. Patrick Stover at Cornell University has suggested that "this may be the best example of a genetic variation that can influence an RDA [recommended dietary allowance] and supports the concept that genetic variation modifies nutrient utilization and potentially dietary requirements."[12]

- Cys282Tyr, an SNP in another gene, has been linked to hereditary hemochromatosis, the iron storage disease that causes iron overload and severe liver damage.

- There are polymorphisms that disrupt alcohol metabolism, lactose metabolism, and liver pathways.

- Some patients who take the antiplatelet drug clopidogrel have a genetic mutation that affects how their liver metabolizes the drug. The drug is less effective in these individuals, and they have a three-fold higher risk of stent thrombosis and death at 1 year.

- Asian people with the genetic variant HLA-B*15:02 may have a life-threatening reaction to the anticonvulsant drug carbamazepine.

- Patients who take abacavir, which is used to treat HIV, are at higher risk of having a hypersensitivity reaction if they carry the HLA-B*5701 gene variant.

Research in pharmacogenomics and nutritional genomics, the branches of medical science that study these personalized reactions to medications and nutrients, is growing. Pharmacogenomics studies have revealed the existence of more than 150 drugs that pose a specific threat to patients with the relevant genetic variants. Among the agents cited by the FDA are common types of drugs, such as statins, antibiotics, antidiabetic drugs, heart medications, and anticoagulants. The list includes pravastatin, propranolol, phenytoin, nortriptyline glyburide, paroxetine, sulfamethoxazole and trimethoprim, tamoxifen, telaprevir, tetrabenazine, thioguanine, thioridazine, trastuzumab, tretinoin, trimipramine, valproic acid, venlafaxine, and warfarin.

The FDA points out that pharmacogenomics can play an important role in identifying responders and nonresponders to medications, preventing adverse events, and optimizing drug dose. Drug labeling may contain information about genomic biomarkers and can describe the following:

- Drug exposure and clinical response variability
- Risk for adverse events
- Genotype-specific dosing
- Drug mechanisms of action

As part of the INTERHEART Study follow-up, Ron Do and associates did research that underscores how genetic individuality affects disease risk and how nutrition can impact that association. They analyzed data from over 8,000 people and compared the health status of 3,820 people with several polymorphisms and 4,294 without the polymorphisms. More specifically, they studied SNPs located on chromosome 9. (Humans have 23 pairs of chromosomes, or 46 in total.) Four SNPs have been found in the p21 section of chromosome 9, each of which increases the risk of heart attack by about 20%. Among individuals who had 2 copies of one of the heart disease-related polymorphisms, there was a twofold increase in risk of heart attack in the INTERHEART Study.

They then compared the dietary patterns of cases and controls and discovered that the risk of heart attack was reduced in people who had one of the SNPs if they consumed a diet that was rich in raw fruits and vegetables. In fact, their risk of heart attack was about the same as in individuals without the genetic mutation when they ate the better diet.[13] Of course, the recommendation to eat more fruits and vegetables is sound advice for everyone and an example of population-based medicine at its best, but many people will ignore the recommendation. Clinicians can bolster that argument if they can show patients with the genetic markers that they are at greater risk of a heart attack when they ignore that admonition.

GENETIC DISEASES MEET GENE EDITING

As we mentioned previously, some diseases are a direct result of specific mutations in our DNA. Sickle cell anemia is one such disease. Until recently, patients with sickle cell anemia had very few treatment options, which didn't do much to relieve their suffering. That started to change with the introduction of a procedure that can correct the genetic flaw in many patients.

If you've kept up with the medical news in the last few years, you're probably familiar with CRISPR, which stands for Clustered Regularly Interspaced Short Palindromic Repeats. The National Human Genomic Institute provides a relatively simple explanation: It's a technology that research scientists use to selectively modify the DNA of living organisms. CRISPR was adapted for use in the laboratory from naturally occurring genome editing systems found in bacteria. What's revolutionary about this technology is that it enables scientists and clinicians to modify the genes in our cells, and in some cases, correct mutations responsible for specific diseases. One of the most dramatic examples of its medical application is in sickle cell anemia.

Sickle cell anemia can cause severe pain and life-threatening complications, and it affects about 72,000 Americans and 1 in 500 Americans of African ancestry or who identify as Black. It's caused by a genetic defect, a mutation in one of the genes required to create hemoglobin. That mutation, in turn, causes a person's red blood cells to take on a sickle-like shape, which makes it difficult for them to travel through the bloodstream, thus blocking small vessels and depriving cells of oxygen and nutrients.

Gene therapy for sickle cell anemia involves extracting an individual's hemoglobin-forming stem cells, using CRISPR to edit the defective gene, and reinfusing the stem cells back into the patient's body. The treatment is life-altering for patients who have suffered from the disease for decades, but it's also very expensive and comes with significant risks, including infection, mouth sores, nausea, vomiting, hair loss, cancer, and infertility.

Sickle cell anemia is only one of many monogenetic diseases that are being treated with this gene therapy. As their name implies, each of these disorders is caused by a single genetic defect, whereas more common disorders are caused by numerous mutations, plus various environmental factors. Some monogenetic disorders are being treated with an approach that differs from CRISPR editing. Severe hemophilia A, for instance, is being treated by linking a corrective gene to a virus, which is then injected into the patient. The result is an increase in levels of factor VIII, which is key for blood clotting and lacking in patients with hemophilia A. As you might expect, gene therapy for hemophilia A is very expensive and comes with a list of possible adverse effects.

FIXING THE GENOME IS NOT THE WHOLE SOLUTION

The genetic breakthroughs we've discussed have given many people hope and transformed their lives, but they're useful for only a very small percentage of patients. They get a lot of publicity, but that shouldn't draw our attention away from all the other "omics" that affect a person's health and risk of disease.

The term "omics" refers to the many biological factors that influence our physical and mental health. Genomics, for example, is the study of the genome. There are other omics, such as proteomics and metabolomics, but the focus of our discussion here is going to be on the intestinal microbiome, which is the microbial content or flora in the human intestinal tract. Understanding the microbiome can contribute to personalized care.

Scientists have been interested in the role of intestinal flora in health and disease for centuries. In the 19th century, for example, Elie Metchnikoff at the Pasteur Institute believed that lactic acid-producing bacteria in the gastrointestinal tract protected humans from disease and that other microbes produced toxic compounds, such as ammonia, that contributed to disease. More recently, investigators have begun to study the role of microorganisms on the surface of the body and inside it to determine how they interact with food, drugs, and a variety of metabolites.

Humans share several types of bacteria. The human gut contains Firmicutes, Bacteroidetes, Proteobacteria, Actinobacteria, Verrucomicrobia, and Fusobacteria. What distinguishes individuals from one another is the wide variation in relative abundance of these bacteria in their intestines. Those differences are evident even in an experimental population of healthy young adults. The microorganisms in your gut can have a significant impact on your biochemical makeup. Metabolism of intestinal bacteria produces by-products such as hippuric acid. High levels of hippuric acid have been implicated in obesity, diabetes, and inflammatory bowel disease. Illustrating the role of the microbiome in establishing one's biochemical individuality, research on healthy adults has found that levels of hippuric acid vary substantially from person to person and over time.[14] Similarly, levels of hippuric acid in urine seem to vary among ethnic groups. Japanese people, for example, have significantly lower levels of the acid in their urine than other groups.

Equally important is the observation that drugs can interact with intestinal microbes, resulting in subtherapeutic and supratherapeutic effects. Simvastatin, which is used to treat high cholesterol, interacts with secondary bile acids in the intestines. Because of that, the drug's ability to lower LDL cholesterol varies from person to person. Animal studies also suggest that suppressing intestinal microbes in the Firmicutes family of bacteria and increasing the dominance of Bacteroidetes can alter the effects of the antipsychotic olanzapine. And there's mounting evidence to suggest that the mechanism of action of the popular antidiabetic agent metformin may depend, in part, on its interaction with gut bacteria.

MAYO CLINIC'S TAPESTRY STUDY

To better understand how genetics and all the other omics influence an individual's health, Mayo Clinic has undertaken a massive, ongoing research project called the Tapestry study. The Center for Individualized Medicine launched it in 2020, under the leadership of Konstantinos Lazaridis, MD. The clinical study is collecting information about how sequencing a patient's DNA could impact their healthcare. The researchers also are developing and improving ways to incorporate genomic information from DNA sequencing into the electronic medical record to create a more complete "Health Tapestry" for each participant in the study.

Sequencing a patient's DNA can uncover genetic variants, some of which determine an individual's risk for disease development. That information could be used to help prevent disease, diagnose it earlier, or provide a patient with more effective therapy. According to the National Library of Medicine database on clinical trials, the study has several broad objectives:[15]

- To detect and compare the actionable genetic findings derived from whole exome sequencing (WES) testing and examine their frequency and association with family history using a large cohort of patients seen across specialties within the Mayo Clinic enterprise. (For an explanation of exome sequencing, see the TechStop on page 112.)

- To assess the effect of actionable genetic findings of patients on healthcare utilization, and patients' acceptance.

- To create a unique vertically integrated data asset (Mayo Clinic Health Tapestry) that links genomics and other omics information to traditional health parameters in the electronic medical record with the aim of elucidating disease formation and outcomes.

- To assess the frequency of hereditary cancer predisposition genes (*BRCA1*, *BRCA2*, Lynch syndrome mismatch repair [MMR] genes) through population screening using WES and the uptake of genetic counseling.

- To study the genetic predisposition to coronavirus disease 2019 (COVID-19) disease, the team proposes using a COVID-19 survey.

As of July 31, 2024, 100,000 patients were enrolled in the Tapestry study. The results are likely to have a major impact on how doctors and patients view genetic testing. So far, over 62,000 exome sequences have been uploaded to the Mayo Clinic Cloud, and more than 1.1 million genetic results have been entered into patients' electronic medical records. Among the discoveries from the gene sequencing were 1,819 mutations, 1.9% of which were disease-related, meaning that patients who carried them are at high risk of rare forms of cancer and elevated cholesterol levels.

What are WES and whole genome sequencing?

The complete genomic information within a sample or individual is known as the whole genome. Exons are the genome's protein-coding regions and are collectively known as the exome. Although the exome is only 2% of the whole genome, it encodes most known disease-related variants.

DNA sequencing—or determination of the order of DNA building blocks (nucleotides) in an individual's genetic code—has advanced the study of genetics and is one of the techniques used to test for genetic disorders. Two methods, WES and whole genome sequencing, are increasingly used in healthcare and research to identify genetic variations; both methods rely on new technologies that allow rapid sequencing of large amounts of DNA. These approaches are known as next-generation sequencing.

The original sequencing technology, called Sanger sequencing, helped scientists determine the human genetic code, but it's time-consuming and expensive. The Sanger method is now automated to make it faster, and it is still in use in laboratories for sequencing short pieces of DNA, but sequencing all of a person's DNA (known as the genome) with it would take years. Next-generation sequencing, in contrast, takes only days or weeks and costs less.

With next-generation sequencing, it's feasible to sequence large amounts of DNA, such as all the pieces of an individual's DNA that provide instructions for making proteins. Known as exon sequencing, this method makes it possible to identify variations in the protein-coding

In a published study that evaluated the Tapestry study results, N. Jewel Samadder and associates found 550 carriers of disease-related genes, including *BRCA1* and *BRCA2*. More importantly, 39% of these people would probably never have been tested for these genetic defects because they didn't meet the criteria for testing from the National Comprehensive Cancer Network.[16]

region of any gene, rather than only a select few genes. Because most known mutations that cause disease occur in exons, WES is thought to be an efficient way to identify possible disease-causing mutations.

DNA variations outside the exons also can affect gene activity and protein production and lead to genetic disorders—variations that WES would miss. Another method, called whole genome sequencing, determines the order of all the nucleotides in an individual's DNA and can identify variations in any part of the genome.

While many more genetic changes can be identified with whole exome and whole genome sequencing than with select gene sequencing, the significance of much of this information is unknown. Because not all genetic changes affect health, it's hard to know whether identified variants are involved in the condition of interest. Sometimes, an identified variant is associated with a different genetic disorder that hasn't yet been diagnosed (these are called incidental or secondary findings).

Besides their use in the clinic, whole exome and whole genome sequencing also are used by researchers. Continued study of exome and genome sequences can help determine whether new genetic variations are associated with health conditions, which will aid disease diagnosis in the future. Polygenic risk scores, which incorporate several SNPs across the genome for disease detection, are the most recent approach.[17] At present, even in research studies that employ sequencing, there's little standardization in the way the techniques are performed.

Based on the evidence we've discussed, it's clear that we're really on the cusp of an era of astonishing innovation—the limits of which aren't even clear yet. By customizing lifestyle interventions and taking into account genetic risk factors—and in rare circumstances, editing genes—we're beginning to see a future that addresses the needs of patients who haven't benefited from the one-size-fits-all approach to healthcare. What remains to be seen is whether this new paradigm will be applied to all segments of society, including people who've previously been excluded because of race, gender, or socioeconomic status.

KEY TAKEAWAYS

- The one-size-fits-all approach to healthcare that you're probably receiving is being replaced by a more personalized approach that takes into account your genetic makeup, unique body chemistry, and lifestyle choices.

- Genetic mutations influence the way individuals respond to medication. Some mutations can cause you to develop unexpected medication side effects. It's now possible to test to see if you're at risk of a genetic/drug interaction.

- Genetic variations can increase a person's nutritional needs, which in turn may change the recommended daily requirement for specific vitamins and minerals.

References

|1| Wallace-Wells D. Suddenly, it looks like we're in a golden age for medicine. *New York Times Magazine*. June 23, https://www.nytimes.com/2023/06/23 /magazine/golden-age-medicine-biomedical-innovation.html.

|2| Schork NJ. Personalized medicine: Time for one-person trials. *Nature*. 2015;530:609-611. doi: 10.1038/520609a.

|3| Cerrato P, Halamka J. *Realizing the Promise of Precision Medicine*. Academic Press/Elsevier; 2018.

|4| Sussman JB, Kent DM, Nelson JP, Hayward RA. Improving diabetes prevention with benefit based tailored treatment: Risk based reanalysis of Diabetes Prevention Program. *BMJ*. 2015;350:h454. doi: 10.1136/bmj.h454.

| 5 | Knowler WC, Barrett-Connor E, Fowler SE, et al. Reduction in the incidence of type 2 diabetes with lifestyle intervention or metformin. *N Engl J Med.* 2002;346:393-403. doi: 10.1056/NEJMoa012512.

| 6 | Roemmich JN, Feda DM, Seelbinder AM, et al. Stress-induced cardiovascular reactivity and atherogenesis in adolescents. *Atherosclerosis.* 2011;215(2):465-470. doi: 10.1016/j.atherosclerosis.2010.12.030.

| 7 | Smyth JM, Ockenfels MC, et al. Individual differences in the diurnal cycle of cortisol. *Psychoneuroendocrinology.* 1997 Feb;22(2):89-105. doi: 10.1016/s0306-4530(96)00039-x.

| 8 | Gildea JJ, Lahiff DT, Van Sciver RE, et al. A linear relationship between the ex-vivo sodium mediated expression of two sodium regulatory pathways as a surrogate marker of salt sensitivity of blood pressure in exfoliated human renal proximal tubule cells: The virtual renal biopsy. *Clin Chim Acta.* 2013 Jun 5:236-242. doi: 10.1016/j.cca.2013.02.021.

| 9 | Felder RA, White MJ, et al. Diagnostic tools for hypertension and salt sensitivity testing. *Curr Opin Nephrol Hypertens.* 2013;22(1):65-76. doi: 10.1097/MNH.0b013e32835b3693.

| 10 | Suhre K, Raffler J, Kastenmüller G. Biochemical insights from population studies with genetics and metabolomics. *Arch Biochem Biophys.* 2016;589:168-176. doi: 10.1016/j.abb.2015.09.023.

| 11 | Beebe K, Kennedy AD. Sharpening precision medicine by a thorough interrogation of metabolic individuality. *Comput Struct Biotechnol J.* 2016;14:97-105. doi: 10.1016/j.csbj.2016.01.001.

| 12 | Stover PJ. Influence of human genetic variation on nutritional requirements. *Am J Clin Nutr.* 2006;83(2):436S-442S. doi: 10.1093/ajcn/83.2.436S.

| 13 | Do R, Xie C, Zhang X, Männistö, Harald K, et al. The effect of chromosome 9p21 variants on cardiovascular disease may be modified by dietary intake: Evidence from a case/control and a prospective study. *PLoS Med.* 2011;8(10):e1001106. doi: 10.1371/journal.pmed.1001106.

| 14 | Patterson AD, Turnbaugh PJ. Microbial determinants of biochemical individuality and their impact on toxicology and pharmacology. *Cell Metab.* 2014;20(5):761-768. doi: 10.1016/j.cmet.2014.07.002.

| 15 | National Library of Medicine. ClinicalTrials.gov. DNA sequencing in clinical practice, Mayo Clinic Health Tapestry study. Accessed August 14, 2024. https://clinicaltrials.gov/study/NCT05212428.

| 16 | Samadder N, Gay E, et al. Exome sequencing identifies carriers of the autosomal dominant cancer predisposition disorders beyond current practice guideline recommendations. *JCO Precis Oncol.* 2024 Jul 8:e2400106. doi: 10.1200/PO.24.00106.

| 17 | National Library of Medicine. MedlinePlus. What are whole exome sequencing and whole genome sequencing? Accessed August 20, 2024. https://medlineplus.gov/genetics/understanding/testing/sequencing/.

CHAPTER 7

We *can't* ignore the social determinants of health

You may be unfamiliar with the term "social determinants of health" (SDOH), sometimes referred to as social drivers of health, suggesting that these factors can be overcome. Unfortunately, until recently, many healthcare professionals also overlooked it. According to the U.S. Department of Health and Human Services,[1] SDOH are the conditions in the environments where people are born, live, learn, work, play, worship, and age that affect a wide range of health, functioning, and quality of life outcomes and risks. SDOH fall into five interrelated domains:

- Economic stability
- Education access and quality
- Healthcare access and quality
- Neighborhood and built environment
- Social and community context

If you have any doubts about the impact of socioeconomic factors on a population's physical health, consider the history of tuberculosis (TB). In 1900, about 200 people per 100,000 died of tuberculosis in the United States, but by 1944, that number had dropped to 50 per 100,000. That change came about despite a lack of readily available treatment or vaccine for TB and was due to significant improvements in living conditions, better nutrition, and a more advanced public health response. In other words, socioeconomic transformation had a positive effect. As one report pointed out: "Improved nutrition probably played an outsized role as macronutrient and micronutrient deficiencies can blunt adaptive and innate immune responses and alter the inflammatory milieu, which leaves hosts vulnerable to *Mycobacterium tuberculosis* and its most severe consequences."[2]

For decades, the healthcare community has focused its efforts almost exclusively on patients' signs and symptoms and the results of their physical examinations and lab tests. But that information doesn't tell the whole story about an individual's medical problems.

We've written often about SDOH, a problem that continues to challenge healthcare policy makers and bedside clinicians alike. In a *New York Times* article,[3] Nicholas Kristof described the profession's inability to adequately address the issue as "the scandal that is American Health Care." His statistics certainly justify this indictment:

- The average person in Mississippi won't make it past age 72, but if they lived in Bangladesh, their average life expectancy would be 72.4 years.

- Life expectancy in Alabama, Arkansas, Kentucky, and Louisiana is less than 74 years, but people living in Japan, Australia, and South Korea typically live to age 84 or beyond.

- Newborns in India, Rwanda, and Venezuela have a longer life expectancy than Native American newborns.

- About 150,000 toe, foot, and leg amputations are performed in the United States each year, making us "a world leader" in that type of surgery. The reason for most of these procedures is poorly managed diabetes.

These troubling statistics are inconsistent with the amount of money the United States invests in healthcare. According to the Bloomberg Prognosis newsletter, every year, our nation spends about $4.3 trillion on it—or about twice as much as other wealthy countries. Many factors contribute to this American scandal, but SDOH plays a major role.

Addressing SDOH issues will require systemic changes in national policies and an attitude adjustment by decision-makers nationwide. Clinicians and the public also can take steps that will make an impact.

Recently, healthcare providers have become much more aware of the impact of social factors on their patients' health, and they've attempted to address these problems. Many of them have come to realize that clinical outcomes will never improve if underlying issues related to SDOH aren't fixed. For example, it's unreasonable to expect a patient to lower their hemoglobin A1c levels—a measure of blood glucose (sugar) levels over 2 to 3 months—if they can't afford the medication prescribed for it. The same goes for asking someone to come to a clinic appointment when they haven't got reliable transportation, or scolding a person whose only source of food is a convenience store for eating highly processed foods rather than fresh fruit and vegetables. In situations like these, many clinicians refer patients to community-based nonprofit organizations. That's helpful, but some clinicians are moving beyond that to more direct intervention. Rahul Vanjani, MD, at Brown University, and associates suggest it may be time for physicians to serve as "street-level bureaucrats."

Vanjani and colleagues point out that many social resources can be tapped with the help of a physician's direct input and signature. They cite the case of a diabetic patient living with his mother in subsidized housing for which only she appeared to be eligible. If the situation didn't change and she died, he was in danger of becoming homeless. But the patient, too, was eligible for the housing. All it took to prove that and ensure that he could remain in his mother's apartment was for his physician to spend 3 minutes printing out and signing a federal form, a U.S. Department of Housing and Urban Development (HUD) Verification of Disability. The authors point out that many clinicians don't know anything about the "often untapped power of medical documentation. . . . A lack of adequate paperwork is often used to justify denial of social services for which people are otherwise eligible, and clinicians can help patients get the necessary paperwork to document medical eligibility for services such as disability housing, prevention of utilities shut-off, disability income, improvement of housing conditions, prevention of incarceration, waiving of court fines and fees, and more."[4]

Of course, fixing social problems is only part of the solution to the troubles facing American healthcare. Our ecosystem devotes far too many resources to the treatment of late-stage disease and far too little to prevention and early detection. One study found that early detection of cancer would save $26 billion per year in the United States. Several digital solutions are emerging to make early detection more readily available to clinicians and patients. For instance, an artificial intelligence (AI)-based algorithm called Sybil, designed to predict risk of lung cancer, has been validated on three independent datasets and has the potential to identify individuals at risk based on a single low-dose chest computed tomography scan.[5]

At Mayo Clinic Platform, we've spent the last several years developing similar digital tools to improve early disease detection. We've also devoted many resources to looking more closely at social factors that interfere with disease prevention and treatment. The financier Warren Buffett once said: "Predicting rain doesn't matter. Building arks does." Even the most impressive algorithm is relatively useless if it doesn't allow us to build better "arks" to address the medical disorder or complications that a digital tool identifies. And building the best healthcare interventions requires that clinicians don't just identify the right signs, symptoms, and biomarkers, whether they are high cholesterol levels, elevated hemoglobin A1c, or a lump in a breast. They also need to understand what's happening in patients' everyday lives outside the clinic—SDOH—and then use those data to inform treatment.

Health professionals are slowly beginning to realize that we can't "remove health and illness from the social contexts in which they are produced," says Simukai Chigudu, Oxford Department of International Development, University of Oxford.[6] That raises questions: What social issues are most likely to influence patients' clinical course and what can be done about them? How can AI help alleviate the impact of these issues?

The Centers for Disease Control and Prevention (CDC) has numerous data sources to help incorporate SDOH into public health initiatives and medical practice. But as the agency points out, moving from data to action is the hard part. The CDC has several programs designed to focus clinicians' attention on key social issues, including socioeconomic status, educational level, and work history. One initiative, for instance, zeroes in on the role of electronic health records (EHRs). Its purpose is to support the incorporation and use of structured work information into health information technology (IT) systems.

How might this SDOH element inform a physician's diagnosis? Consider a man with hypertension (high blood pressure) who doesn't respond to a low-sodium diet or medication. Awareness of his 10-year history as a house-painter might point the clinician in the direction of lead poisoning, a possible cause of hypertension. Similarly, an advanced practice provider might be at a loss as to why a woman with type 2 diabetes has had a spike in hemoglobin A1c levels. She works a night shift, which can affect diabetes control. Wouldn't it be helpful if the EHR system could throw up a flag about that connection and provide recommendations for diabetes management among shift workers?

The CDC is creating a data model that incorporates work information, as well as national standards for vocabulary, system interoperability, and instructions for health IT system developers.

At Mayo Clinic, we're also studying the impact of SDOH on health and disease. Young Juhn, MD, MPH, director of the AI Program and Precision Population Science Lab of the Department of Pediatric and Adolescent Medicine at Mayo Clinic, has studied the effects of socioeconomic status on health since 2006. With support from the National Institutes of Health (NIH), he developed and validated a housing-based socioeconomic measure called the housing-based socioeconomic status index (HOUSES), which is being used by researchers to help understand health disparities and differences in a variety of health outcomes in both adults and children. The index has enabled researchers to overcome the absence of socioeconomic measures in commonly used data sources (e.g., medical records or administrative data), conduct geospatial analysis in health disparities research, and apply a life-course approach.

The HOUSES index is an objective way to measure the individual-level socioeconomic status of patients because it's based on real property data for individual (not aggregated) housing units and derived from public records. It uses four data points: the number of bedrooms in a person's residence, the number of bathrooms, square footage of the unit, and estimated building value of the unit. The index can help target patients who are most at risk of poor health outcomes and inadequate access to healthcare, demonstrating the real value of adding SDOH into the mix by addressing limitations of the existing SDOH. For example, one study showed that patients with a higher HOUSES score (quartiles 2-4) had a 53% lower risk of kidney transplant rejection than those with the lowest score.[7] Dr. Juhn and his colleagues found that HOUSES can predict 44 different health outcomes and behavioral risk factors in adults and children.

Of course, clinicians still have to be reasonable about their expectations. Even if an algorithm were outfitted with every conceivable SDOH, it still might not reduce disparities in healthcare. For example, a patient and their clinician could choose to ignore an improved algorithm's recommendation for a diagnostic test because it's too expensive, the patient can't get to the testing facility, or the patient doesn't see the value of the test.

ADDRESSING HEALTH INEQUITIES

Housing is only one of many socioeconomic factors that affect a person's health and impact their access to healthcare. The availability of high-speed internet access and cloud computing services are other factors to consider. In fact, reliable access to the internet is sometimes called a "super determinant" of health. The U.S. federal government states: "Internet access is increasingly recognized as a 'super determinant' of health. It plays a role in health care outcomes and influences more traditionally recognized social determinants of health, such as education, employment, and healthcare access. The Federal Communications Commission (FCC) estimates that 19 million people in the United States lack access to reliable high-speed broadband internet. This phenomenon is known as the digital divide and has focused on rural areas and pockets of segregated urban areas [that] are also disconnected."[8]

This digital divide can have serious repercussions for a patient's health. Lack of fast broadband internet service increases the time it takes to get prompt medical attention and often makes it impossible to use telemedicine services. As you might expect, people in poorer neighborhoods are much more likely to face this technological hurdle. By one estimate, about 8 in 10 households with incomes above $100,000 have high-speed internet, compared with 5 in 10 households with incomes below $25,000, based on 2021 data.[8]

The COVID pandemic made it obvious to many of us that broadband-enabled telemedicine services can have a major impact on healthcare. A 2022 review of 28 studies found that telehealth services were effective in managing physical and mental health problems, including depression, diabetes, and hypertension. They also improved access to care by "providing financial and time benefits to patients." But the report also showed that such services were problematic for people because of "cost and limited digital and health literacy."[9] Unfortunately, the expanded access to high-speed internet that was put into place during the pandemic may disappear because the Affordable Connectivity Program (ACP) ended in April 2024. It was part of the Infrastructure Investment and Jobs Act, which Congress passed in 2021 to make high-speed online service more affordable. Since then, more than 23 million low-income households have benefited from the $14 billion allocated by the ACP to support high-speed access.[10] Through the ACP, eligible households could get a discount of up to $30 per month toward internet service. For households on qualifying tribal lands, the discount was up to $75 per month.

Households were also eligible to receive a one-time discount of up to $100 to purchase a laptop, desktop computer, or tablet from participating providers if they contributed more than $10 and less than $50 toward the purchase price.

In the absence of a federal program, individual states can help close the digital divide with their own programs. A study by the Pew Charitable Trusts of state broadband programs nationwide found that they vary, depending on the local political environment, level of resources available, geography of areas that are unserved or underserved, and the entities that provide broadband service. For example, Colorado, Minnesota, Tennessee, Virginia, and Wisconsin "support broadband deployment in unserved and underserved areas through grant programs that fund a portion of the cost of deployment."[11] Those states also promote "accountability by requiring that grantees demonstrate they are providing the service they were funded to deliver while also providing states with the data needed to evaluate the program and progress toward defined goals."[11] The study highlights promising broadband expansion practices, such as collaborating with state broadband program representatives, internet service providers, local governments, and broadband coalitions. Other practices include stakeholder outreach and engagement, policy framework, planning and capacity building, funding and operations, and program evaluation and evolution. Policymakers and service providers can examine practices in these states and adapt them to fit their needs and contexts to bridge the broadband gap.

PUTTING SPECIAL EMPHASIS ON MENTAL HEALTH

Because mental health is such an important component of SDOH, we want to discuss it in more detail and take a closer look at some of the digital health tools currently being used to address this issue. By one estimate, 1 in 4 people worldwide experience a mental or neurological disorder during their lifetime. And more than 300 million people experience depression.[12] Since the COVID pandemic, those numbers probably have increased as the population has continued to face the economic and personal pressures that began during the outbreak. And because there are too few professionals to meet the need for mental healthcare, many patients are turning to online solutions. The research on these digital tools is mixed, and it's important to differentiate between mobile apps designed to improve your mental health in general and those intended to treat more serious problems, such as clinical depression and anxiety.

Researchers at the University of California, San Francisco (UCSF) evaluated an app called Headspace, which is designed to help people ease stress. They found that "used daily for just 10 minutes, [it] reduced stress in a meaningful way and the benefits lasted for two months after stopping use. Headspace can be done in the morning or evening, alone or with family, or anytime you need to take a break."[13] Other programs that the UCSF authors listed as potentially useful for anxiety and depression included MindShiftCBT (CBT refers to cognitive behavioral therapy) and PTSD Coach, which has been used by patients experiencing post-traumatic stress disorder. PTSD Coach was developed by the U.S. Department of Veterans Affairs National Center for PTSD and the Department of Defense National Center for Telehealth and Technology.

An in-depth analysis of mental health smartphone apps also had positive things to say about these digital tools. The study looked at 176 randomized controlled trials (RCTs). (RCTs are considered the most reliable way to measure the value of a clinical intervention because they compare patients receiving the treatment to a control group of people who aren't given the treatment.) The researchers found: "Apps had overall significant although small effects on symptoms of depression . . . and generalized anxiety . . . as compared to control groups."[14] They concluded that "apps have overall small but significant effects on symptoms of depression and generalized anxiety, and that specific features of apps—such as CBT or mood monitoring features and chatbot technology—are associated with larger effect sizes."

THE LINK BETWEEN EDUCATION AND HEALTH

Education can't be ignored when we're making a list of possible SDOH. Surveys have consistently shown that better educated people are healthier. They're less likely to have high blood pressure, emphysema, or diabetes, for instance. The National Bureau of Economic Research (NBER) points out: "An additional four years of education lowers five-year mortality by 1.8 percentage points; it also reduces the risk of heart disease by 2.16 percentage points, and the risk of diabetes by 1.3 percentage points."[15] In 1999, according to NBER, high school dropouts between the ages of 25 and 64 were more than twice as likely to diet as their peers who had some college education. Why this disparity?

One likely cause is stress. As a general rule, more education translates into higher salaries, although there are many exceptions. And less income is often accompanied by the stress of having to make ends meet. Do you spend your limited resources on groceries, or your prescription medication? How do you get to work in a rural community that has no public transportation system when your car dies and you can't afford to buy a new one? The list of challenges is almost endless. These types of stressors are bound to have an impact on a person's mental and physical health.

It's also likely that better education means more exposure to accurate and timely information about health. The Center on Society and Health, part of Virginia Commonwealth University, summed up this connection:

> In addition to being prepared for better jobs, people with more educa-
> tion are more likely to learn about healthy behaviors. Educated patients
> may be more able to understand their health needs, follow instructions,
> advocate for themselves and their families, and communicate effectively
> with health providers. . . . People who are more educated are more
> receptive to health education campaigns. Education can also lead to
> more accurate health beliefs and knowledge, and thus to better lifestyle
> choices, but also to better skills and greater self-advocacy. Education
> improves skills such as literacy, develops effective habits, and may
> improve cognitive ability. The skills acquired through education can
> affect health indirectly (through better jobs and earnings) or directly
> (through ability to follow health care regimens and manage diseases),
> and they can affect the ability of patients to navigate the health system,
> such as knowing how to get reimbursed by a health plan. Thus, more
> highly educated individuals may be more able to understand health care
> issues and follow treatment guidelines. The quality of doctor-patient
> communication is also poorer for patients of low socioeconomic status.
> A review of the effects of health literacy on health found that people
> with lower health literacy are more likely to use emergency services and
> be hospitalized and are less likely to use preventive services such as
> mammography or take medications and interpret labels correctly.
> Among the elderly, poor health literacy has been linked to poorer health
> status and higher death rates.[16]

Better education also brings with it more critical thinking skills, which in turn make a person less gullible and less easily swayed by outlandish conspiracy theories. Conspiracy beliefs are "assumptions that a group of actors meet in secret agreement in order to pursue goals that are widely seen as malevolent. Such conspiracy theories often implicate powerful groups like governmental institutions (e.g., allegations that 9/11 was an inside job), major branches of industry (e.g., pharmaceutical companies), or ethnic groups that carry negative stereotypes (e.g., Muslims, Jews)."[17] Several studies have linked high education levels with a decreased likelihood that people will believe in such theories.

WE CAN'T IGNORE COMMUNITY

At the beginning of this chapter, we briefly mentioned community context as an SDOH. Having strong bonds with others in one's community is essential to good physical and emotional health. A lack of such connections can have a profound negative impact. Unfortunately, many people don't realize just how harmful social isolation and loneliness can be. As a risk factor, they're about as harmful as smoking 15 cigarettes a day or having an alcohol use disorder. Put another way, social isolation and loneliness increase the risk of dying by 26% and 29%, respectively.[18] On a more positive note, research shows that people who are socially engaged are less likely to experience disability, and their risk of dying is lower.

Amy Freedman and Jennifer Nicolle, two Canadian physicians, illustrate the problem of loneliness and isolation through a patient scenario: Natasha, 85 years old, lost her husband 6 months ago to advanced dementia. She leaves her apartment only to shop for groceries and to visit her doctor. Her adult children live too far away to provide any significant in-person support. And during the long years of caring for her husband, she lost touch with all her friends. How can Natasha, and people like her, be helped?

The first step is to identify them. Not everyone who lives alone and keeps to themselves is by definition lonely or experiencing the harmful effects of social isolation, but many of them are. Relatives, friends, and clinicians need a way to spot these vulnerable people. Studies suggest that family physicians are not very good at identifying them or figuring out what specifically they can do to help. Assessment tools are one approach. A patient can be asked 3 simple questions to find out if they're lonely:

- How often do you feel that you lack companionship?
- How often do you feel left out?
- How often do you feel isolated from others?

There are three responses: hardly ever, some of the time, and often. Higher scores suggest greater loneliness.[18] Each question is given a score of 1 to 3 and then the scores for the three questions are totaled. For instance, if a patient said they often lacked companionship, often felt left out, and often felt isolated, they would be given a score of 9, which strongly suggests the need for intervention.

Solutions for loneliness, especially among the elderly, include social clubs, videoconferencing with family members, online chat rooms, and interactive video games. Psychotherapy is another option, including mindfulness-based stress reduction and reminiscence group therapy. There's also evidence to suggest that pets—even robotic ones—can be a real source of comfort and companionship. Other possibilities are exercise programs that bring the person in touch with others in the community and befriending services that involve volunteers visiting the person or talking with them on the telephone. Drs. Freedman and Nicolle also cite research that suggests that computer and internet training can help lonely elders, probably by giving them the skills needed to interact more effectively with others online.

Digital assistants like Apple's Siri and Amazon's Alexa, too, can help fill the empty hours for those feeling isolated. One of our elderly relatives uses Alexa to get news updates, weather reports, recipes, and the occasional joke. For those with failing eyesight, these services do make a difference. Finally, there are the latest AI-driven chatbots, like ChatGPT, which can have long, realistic-sounding conversations with users. Of course, caution is needed with these generative AI tools because they can be abused.

KEY TAKEAWAYS

- Many social drivers can affect your health, including your education level, your involvement in your community, and your accessibility to medical professionals.

- Many medical professionals are now paying attention to these so-called social determinants of health, asking patients about their everyday lives outside the clinic so that they can create a more personalized healthcare plan.

- Some programs now incorporate social drivers directly into a patient's electronic health record so that others on the medical team can address them.

References

|1| Healthy People 2030: Social determinants of health. U.S. Department of Health and Human Services. Office of Disease Prevention and Health Promotion. Accessed September 4, 2024. https://health.gov/healthypeople/priority-areas /social-determinants-health.

|2| Sinha P, Mehta S. Food: The tuberculosis vaccine we already have. *Lancet.* 2023 Aug 19;402(10402):588-589. doi: 10.1016/S0140-6736(23)01321-1.

|3| Kristof N. How do we fix the scandal that is American Health Care? *New York Times.* August 23, 2023. Accessed September 4, 2024. https://www.nytimes .com/2023/08/16/opinion/health-care-life-expectancy-poverty.html?search ResultPosition=1.

|4| Vanjani R et al. The social determinants of health—moving beyond screen-and-refer to intervention. *New England Journal of Medicine.* 2023 Aug 9;389:569-573. doi: 10.1056/NEJMms2211450.

|5| Mikhael PG, Wohlwend J, Yala A, et al. Sybil: A validated deep learning model to predict future lung cancer risk from a single low-dose chest computed tomography. *J Clin Oncol.* 2023 Apr 20;41(12):2191-2200. doi: 10.1200/JCO.22.01345.

|6| Chigudu S. An ironic guide to colonialism in global health. *Lancet.* 2021;397(10288):1874-1975. doi: 10.1016/S0140-6736(21)01102-8.

|7| Stevens M, Beebe TJ, Wi C-L, et al. HOUSES index as an innovative socioeconomic measure predicts graft failure among kidney transplant recipients. *Transplantation.* 2020 Nov;104(11):2383-2392. doi: 10.1097/TP.00000000 00003131.

|8| Turcios Y. Digital access: A super determinant of health. Substance Abuse and Mental Health Administration. Updated March 22, 2023. Accessed September 10, 2024. https://www.samhsa.gov/blog/digital-access-super-determinant -health.

|9| Truong M, Yeganeh L, Cook O, et al. Using telehealth consultations for health-care provision to patients from non-Indigenous racial/ethnic minorities: A systematic review. *J Am Med Inform Assoc.* 2022 Apr 13;29(5):970-982. doi: 10.1093/jamia/ocac015.

|10| Ashworth B. Millions of Americans might lose internet access today. Here's what you need to know. *Wired*. April 30, 2024. Accessed September 12, 2024. https://www.wired.com/story/affordable-connectivity-program-ending/.

|11| Pew Charitable Trusts. How states are expanding broadband access. Accessed October 15, 2024. https://www.pewtrusts.org/en/research-and-analysis /reports/2020/02/how-states-are-expanding-broadband-access.

|12| Andualem M, Dagmawi K, Alemayehu N. Prevalence and severity of depression and its association with substance use in Jimma Town, Southwest Ethiopia. *Depress Res Treat*. 2016 Mar 16;2016:3460462. doi: 10.1155/2016/3460462.

|13| University of California, San Francisco. Weill Institute for Neurosciences. Department of Psychiatry and Behavioral Sciences. Useful wellness and mental health apps. Accessed September 18, 2024. https://psychiatry.ucsf.edu/coping resources/apps.

|14| Linardon J, Torous J, Firth J, et al. Current evidence on the efficacy of mental health smartphone apps for symptoms of depression and anxiety. A meta-analysis of 176 randomized controlled trials. *World Psychiatry*. 2024 Feb;23(1):139-149. doi: 10.1002/wps.21183.

|15| National Bureau of Economic Research. The Digest. March 1, 2007. The effects of education on health. Accessed September 23, 2024. https://www.nber.org /digest/effects-education-health.

|16| Virginia Commonwealth University. Center on Society and Health. Why education matters to health: Exploring the causes. February 13, 2015. Accessed September 23, 2024. https://societyhealth.vcu.edu/work/the-projects/why -education-matters-to-health-exploring-the-causes.html#gsc.tab=0.

|17| Van Prooijen J-W. Why education predicts decreased belief in conspiracy theories. *Appl Cogn Psychol*. 2017 Jan-Feb;31(1):50-58. doi: 10.1002/acp.3301.

|18| Freedman A, Nicolle J. Social isolation and loneliness: The new geriatric giants. *Can Fam Physician*. 2020 Mar;66(3):176-182.

CHAPTER 8

Generative AI: The next revolution in digital health

If you've ever talked to Apple's Siri, Google Assistant, or Amazon's Alexa, you know how realistic they can sound. Their ability to answer basic questions about the weather, the news of the day, or the latest recipes for apple pie once seemed magical, but most of us now take them for granted. However, none of these chatbots come close to the "magic" of ChatGPT, Bard, Gemini, and several other artificial intelligence (AI)-enabled chatbots that are revolutionizing how humans and computers interact.

Chatbots fall into three broad categories, deriving their ability to talk with us by: 1) relying on a set of rules that link certain keywords in a person's query to prerecorded answers; 2) using a form of AI called machine learning, which creates a response using data they have been trained on; or 3) generating new responses to a person's question by taking advantage of massive amounts of data. This third group uses generative AI. ChatGPT, for instance, is a chatbot that uses generative pre-trained transformers and a specific subgroup called large language models (LLMs). As Google explains it: "A generative model can take what it has learned from the examples it's been shown and create something entirely new based on that information. Hence the word 'generative!' LLMs are one type of generative AI since they generate novel combinations of text in the form of natural-sounding language."[1]

LLMs like ChatGPT have the potential to both benefit and harm users. With that in mind, it makes sense to understand the underlying technology. As the name implies, an LLM uses massive amounts of data, and in the case of text documents, can learn all sorts of linguistic patterns and associations to create a deep knowledge base to draw on. That, in turn, enables the model to make logical predictions about which words, sentences, and paragraphs should follow one another. Nigam Shah, MD, professor of medicine and biomedical data science at Stanford University, has provided an explanation of how these digital tools work.[2]

If we start with a simple sentence like *Where are we going?* and leave out the word "going" and then ask a computer to predict that word, the probability looks like this:

> 66 P(S), the probability of the completed sentence = P of "where" x the P of "are" (given "Where") x P of "we" (given "Where are") x P of ("going" given "Where are we").

The same probability would exist if the training data included a different sentence: *Where are we at?* And if the dataset consisted of only those two sentences, Dr. Shah points out that the probability of correctly predicting the missing word—"going" or "at"—would be 0.5—a 50/50 chance. An LLM learns such probabilities on a massive scale. Datasets of hundreds or thousands of samples typically would be needed to train a predictive model that classifies a skin lesion as melanoma or a normal mole, whereas billions of data points would be used with an LLM. Some technologists speculate that a trillion samples were used to train OpenAI's ChatGPT-4.

To understand how these chatbots work, it helps to deconstruct the term. The term "chat" is pretty obvious. These models talk to users, with words, images, even computer code. GPT stands for Generative Pre-trained Transformer. Chatbots are generative in the sense that they're creating new information, which can be accurate, inaccurate, or a complete fabrication. They're pre-trained because the model deliberately masks some of the words in the training data. Then the partially masked data are inserted into a complex transformer program that uses various encoders and decoders, developed by Google. The chatbot is told to fill in or predict the missing words or data that have been masked.

Of course, none of these technical details touch on the ethical and practical implications of using chatbots in the real world. As we've pointed out in previous publications, chatbots can be used to generate fake videos depicting prominent public figures saying or doing things they never did. They've been used by students to answer test questions, and they've spread all sorts of conspiracy theories. On the plus side, chatbots are also being used to take on routine business tasks, enabling employees to focus on more complex work. Some clinicians are also using chatbots to answer patients' questions or summarize patient histories by extracting key elements from electronic health records (EHRs). The list goes on.

A DEEPER DIVE INTO GENERATIVE AI AND LARGE LANGUAGE MODELS

Many AI systems are designed to address specific tasks, such as classifying data and helping users choose between two options. A neural network that analyzes thousands of images of skin lesions, for instance, can classify some as melanomas and others as benign moles. A decision tree might help clinicians choose between lab test A and lab test B when making a differential diagnosis of a respiratory infection. (A differential diagnosis is a list of the most likely diagnoses.) Generative AI systems can also do these tasks, but they have more capabilities.

LLMs are AI systems that focus on language and collect massive amounts of data to generate new content, which means they're a type of generative AI. However, many LLMs go beyond gathering words from natural language to also collect and analyze computer code, images, and more. ChatGPT, for instance, can generate essays, write code, and draw pictures.

Understanding pre-training

Pre-trained AI models are neural networks, which simulate the brain's network of neurons. An artificial neural network that distinguishes melanoma from a normal mole will be trained on tens of thousands of images to teach itself how to recognize small differences between normal and abnormal skin growths. These "neurons" are nodes or layers that are connected to one another; as each node is excited by data coming from a digital image, those data are sent to the next node. The excitation transferred from one node to the next is represented by a specific number or weight. In the case of the skin cancer algorithm, the excitation is the result of the network analyzing the millions of pixels in each image. Data representing the pixels in an image can be sent through nodes in the first input layer and are then transferred to the next layer, with the strength of each signal indicated by specific numerical values. The goal is to arrive at an output—in this case, a conclusion that the image represents skin cancer or not.[3] But the neural networks in LLMs do much more. In healthcare, they're now being used by clinicians to help improve medical office scheduling or recruit patients for clinical trials. As we explain later in this chapter, some are being tested to see if they can improve the diagnosis of complex diseases.

Using pre-trained models is appealing to app developers because they don't have to do as much training themselves. Instead, they can focus their attention on customizing a model to meet specific needs. Pre-trained models can also save money. Nvidia, which makes the computer chips that run LLMs, explains, "To create such a model from scratch, developers require enormous datasets, often with billions of rows of data. These can be pricey and challenging to obtain, but compromising on data can lead to poor performance of the model."[4]

Several technology companies now offer developers access to pre-trained models, along with the application programing interfaces (APIs) needed to use them. Google Cloud, for example, provides machine learning APIs in a variety of different "flavors," including vision, video, translation, natural language, cloud text-to-speech, and cloud speech-to-text.[5]

At a high level, generative AI systems can analyze a sequence of words that have been input as a "prompt" and create an output or response that sounds like it was generated by an intelligent human. Consider the input sentence in Figure 8.1. It was created with the help of an attention mechanism. As the figure shows, the mechanism reacts to each word, using back propagation to generate additional relevant words. Eventually, an entire story can be created. The process also requires use of a technology called transformers.

Understanding transformers

Amazon Web Services defines a transformer as "a type of neural network architecture that transforms or changes an input sequence into an output sequence."[6] Although there are many types of transformers, the basic architecture includes three components:

- Tokenization
- Embedding layers, which convert tokens into representatively meaningful data with a unique address
- Transformer layers, which include encoders and decoders

Tokens are the basic units to be analyzed by the model, typically a group of characters, such as words plus metadata. For instance, the expression

FIGURE 8.1
How pre-training works

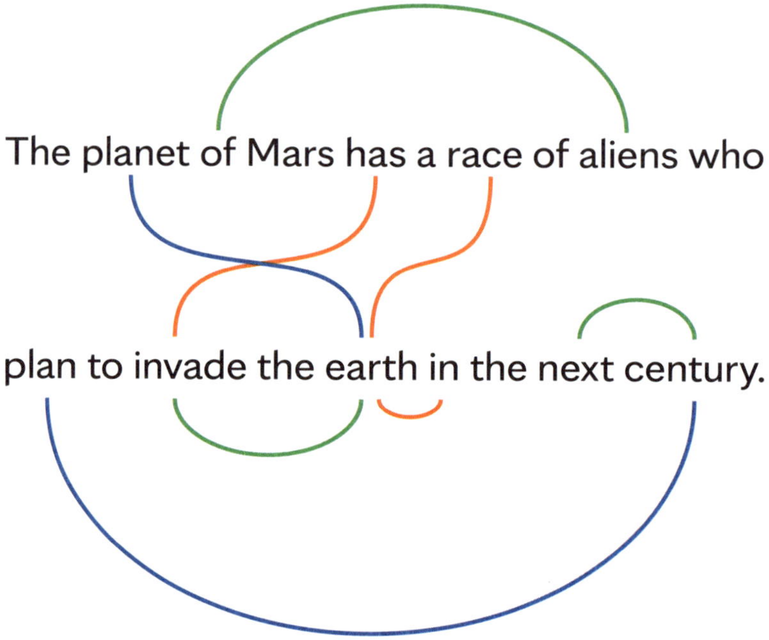

The planet of Mars has a race of aliens who

plan to invade the earth in the next century.

"Hello, how are you today?" contains 16 tokens.[7] Tokenization replaces the plain English content with data elements that can be imported into the embedding software. Neural networks require numbers to represent each word; these are the weights used in the network. But having a numerical representation of the words in the input statement is not enough. The embedding layer must also have a way to tell us what position in the sequence it has relative to the other words. That's done through a position encoding program.[8] The embedding layer is the first step in a GPT model. It depicts the stages in the transformer process, which include the encoders and decoders. Michael Phi provides a more in-depth explanation in the YouTube video "Illustrated Guide to Transformers Neural Network: A Step by Step Explanation."[8]

HOW DOES ALL THIS TECHNOLOGY HELP ME?

At this point, you may be wondering about the practical applications of generative AI and LLMs. Will they help your physician provide you with better care and improve your experience as a patient? Considering that there were three promising healthcare applications of chatbots as this book went to press, the answer is yes.

Improving communication with patients

One of the problems clinicians have is coping with the mountain of emails they receive from patients. Some of them require an immediate direct reply, but others are less urgent and may benefit from AI assistance. Recent studies suggest that generative AI can help craft these messages, saving clinicians time and speeding up communication with patients. In one experiment, 52 physicians used AI-generated replies to patient queries. The researchers found "increased message read time, no change in reply time, and significantly longer replies. Physicians valued AI-generated drafts as a compassionate starting point for their replies and also noted areas for improvement."[9] The questions examined during the study were focused on prescription refills, test results, paperwork, and general questions. The generative AI (GenAI) replies did speed up communication, but the researchers found differences between email replies from actual doctors and the AI-generated ones that were reviewed by doctors before being sent: "While both replies demonstrated a caring attitude to the patient's concerns, the physician's reply contained greater details regarding medication concerns and offered a more collaborative approach to decision-making regarding further laboratory testing. The physician retained the pleasantries in the GenAI draft and made many substantive changes."

So, realistic-sounding chatbots may save clinicians time answering patients' questions, but there's a downside to consider. In a recent editorial, one physician welcomed the use of these tools because at least one study suggested that chatbot-written emails are more empathetic than those written by clinicians. His reaction to that news was: "In the end, it doesn't actually matter if doctors feel compassion or empathy toward patients; it only matters if they act like it. In much the same way, it doesn't matter that AI has no idea what we, or it, are even talking about. There are linguistic formulas for human empathy and compassion, and we should not hesitate to use good ones, no matter who—or what—is the author."[10] But that perspective overlooks one important fact: Patients can often tell the difference between genuine compassion and empathy and the canned version that comes from a machine, or even a clinician following a script. Sincerity is not easily faked, and it depends not just on the *words* you choose but on the intonation of your voice, the expression on your face, your body language, and your emotions. ChatGPT has yet to duplicate that.

Other researchers have focused on the accuracy of GenAI answers to patients' questions. For instance, one group of scientists tested ChatGPT, Bard, and Bing to see if the tools would give correct answers to questions about vasectomy. The AI responses were graded on a scale of 1 to 4 on clarity, accuracy, and evidence-based information. ChatGPT averaged 1.367 (1 is the highest score), Bard 2.167, and Bing 1.8.[11]

As we said earlier, an oft-quoted study that compared AI algorithms' answers to patients' questions with answers from doctors concluded that ChatGPT's answers were more accurate and more empathetic.[12] A closer look at that research underscores its limitations. The judges for the competition were a panel of three medical professionals who rated the answers. As one critic pointed out: "The evaluators applied untested, subjective criteria for quality and empathy. Importantly, they did not assess *actual accuracy* of the answers. Nor were answers assessed for fabrication, a problem that has been noted with ChatGPT."[13]

Chatbots and medical diagnosis and treatment

One of the most important questions we need to answer about chatbots is whether they can improve medical diagnosis and treatment. To address the issue, it helps to first understand the foundation upon which chatbots are built. For decades, innovators have been looking for ways to use computer technology to improve patient care and ease clinicians' workloads. Some experts have even suggested that AI-based algorithms are as effective as physicians in diagnosing specific diseases. In 2016, Varun Gulshan at Google and his associates from several medical schools tested that theory, using an artificial neural network (ANN) to analyze retinal images.[14] (An ANN mimics the human brain's network of nerve cells and can process data through a series of nodes that are similar to the neurons in the brain.) The researchers used the ANN to look for evidence of diabetic retinopathy, a common eye complication that causes blindness in many diabetics and found that its diagnostic skills were on par with those of several board-certified ophthalmologists. Since then, additional research has been done to determine if similar digital tools can augment or replace clinicians.

For example, British and German investigators analyzed 82 studies that compared deep learning algorithms with clinicians to determine their respective abilities to detect diseases by using medical images.[15] They "found the diagnostic performance of deep learning models to be equivalent to that of health care professionals. However, a major finding of the review is that few studies presented externally validated results or compared the performance of deep learning models and health care professionals using the same sample." A second analysis from British and American researchers also compared AI with clinicians, concluding: "Few prospective deep learning studies and randomized trials exist in medical imaging. Most nonrandomized trials are not prospective, are at high risk of bias, and deviate from existing reporting standards. Data and code availability are lacking in most studies, and human comparator groups are often small."[16]

Now that ChatGPT and other LLMs have emerged, many thought leaders are also wondering how they'll perform when challenged with diagnostic puzzles. With that in mind, we sent ChatGPT-4 the following prompt:

> 66 Mr. Jones, 59 years old, with a history of hypertension, stroke, and elevated lipid levels, arrives in the ED complaining of sudden-onset intense substernal chest pain that radiates to his left leg but does not affect his left arm or jaw. He also has an elevated troponin I, an enzyme that suggests damage to the heart muscle or myocardium. What is the correct diagnosis?

ChatGPT replied:

> 66 Based on the symptoms and medical history provided, Mr. Jones is presenting with a potential myocardial infarction (MI), also known as a heart attack. The sudden onset of intense chest pain just below the breastbone that radiates to his left leg is a common symptom of a heart attack. The fact that the pain does not affect his left arm or jaw is not unusual, as some heart attacks can present with atypical symptoms.
>
> The elevated troponin I level is also a significant finding, as it indicates damage to the heart muscle. Troponin is a protein released into the bloodstream when heart muscle cells are damaged or die, which is a hallmark of a heart attack. It is important to note that a definitive diagnosis can only be made by a healthcare professional after conducting a thorough medical evaluation, including a physical examination, ECG, and other tests as necessary. Prompt medical attention is essential in suspected cases of heart attack, as early intervention can improve outcomes and reduce the risk of complications.

Several years ago, a case report published in the *Journal of General Internal Medicine* described an identical patient scenario in which J. William

Schleifer, MD, and colleagues at the University of Alabama in Birmingham explained their diagnostic reasoning and the conclusion they reached. We provided a shortened version of that case in one of our recent books, *Reinventing Clinical Decision Support: Data Analysis, Artificial Intelligence, and Diagnostic Reasoning*. Based on a methodical review of all the patient data, Dr. Schleifer and his colleagues questioned the significance of the patient's radiating left leg pain. One of the hallmarks of a genuine expert diagnostician is their more completely developed disease scripts and their ability to spot inconsistencies that don't fit into these scripts. The leg pain was one of those clues that might warrant a walk down a different diagnostic path.

They also used a reasoning technique sometimes referred to as pre-mortem examination. Essentially, they asked themselves: What would happen once a specific diagnosis is made and acted upon? What are the consequences, good and bad? In the case of Mr. Jones, if he were treated with the anticoagulants usually indicated for a typical MI but he actually had another condition, such as a ruptured aorta, the consequences could prove disastrous. The pre-mortem analysis and the fact that the patient had radiating left leg pain were enough to postpone treating the alleged MI until additional data were collected. Once the patient was admitted to the medical floor, the appearance of a systolic murmur plus chest pain strongly suggested an aortic dissection, a tear in this major blood vessel; the tear was finally confirmed with a computed tomography (CT) angiogram. The imaging study also documented that the dissection extended all the way down Mr. Jones's thoracic descending aorta, which explained the mysterious leg pain.

Their correct diagnosis raises the question: Why didn't ChatGPT reach the same conclusion? The scenario dramatically illustrates the difference between LLMs trained on the general content of the internet and the "database" residing within the brain of a veteran cardiologist with decades of clinical experience and expert reasoning skills. It also underscores that LLMs don't actually reason, at least not in the way humans do, including using critical thinking skills that computers have yet to master. As Chrag Shah at the University of Washington explains, "Language models are not knowledgeable beyond their ability to capture patterns of strings or words and spit them out in a probabilistic manner. . . . It gives the false impression of intelligence."[17]

Admittedly, the chatbot did warn users that a definitive diagnosis wasn't possible and should only be made by a healthcare professional "after conducting a thorough medical evaluation, including a physical examination, ECG, and other tests as necessary." But realistically, many patients, and perhaps a few clinicians, will rely heavily on its conclusion, with potentially life-threatening consequences.

Some medical experts have said that our test of ChatGPT may not have been fair. There are many other, more sophisticated ways to use ChatGPT, rather than directly asking it to make a diagnosis, and several researchers have explored these options to evaluate an LLM's ability to do clinical reasoning. Hidde ten Berg and associates, for instance, did a retrospective analysis of 30 emergency department (ED) patients and asked ChatGPT to generate a differential diagnosis for each patient based on the notes that a physician had entered into the EHR during their initial ED presentation. The chatbot's responses were compared with the physicians' diagnoses. Using the patients' medical histories and physician exams, clinicians "correctly included the diagnosis in the top differential diagnoses for 83% of cases," compared with 87% for ChatGPT-4.[18] When lab results were included in the analysis, the clinicians' accuracy increased to 87%, whereas ChatGPT-4's remained at 87%.

Other researchers have presented ChatGPT with 36 patient scenarios extracted from the *Merck Manual of Diagnosis and Therapy,* using an iterative prompting approach. The chatbot was initially asked to create a differential diagnosis and then review diagnostic testing, make a final diagnosis, and recommend treatment. ChatGPT had an overall accuracy of 71.7% across all 36 clinical vignettes, with its strongest performance in making a final diagnosis (76.9%) versus 60.3% for the initial differential diagnosis.[19]

Still other investigators have evaluated ChatGPT's ability to serve as a clinical decision support system (CDSS). They reviewed the medical histories of six geriatric patients whose definitive diagnosis had been delayed by more than a month. The patients' presentations were given to ChatGPT-4 and a commercially available CDSS (Isabel Healthcare) for analysis. The chatbot was not informed of the clinicians' final diagnosis. ChatGPT-4 accurately diagnosed 4 of 6 patients (66.7%), clinicians 2 of 6 (33.3%), and Isabel 0.[20] The investigators discovered that certain key words helped determine how accurate the chatbot was in making the diagnosis, including "abdominal aortic aneurysm," "proximal stiffness," "acid-fast bacilli in urine," and "metronidazole."

Studies like these have prompted some clinicians to assert that LLMs are capable of deep reasoning and logical thinking, concluding: "Rather than competing with conventional information sources such as search engines, databases, Wikipedia, research articles, reviews, or textbooks, LLMs offer an entirely new means of information processing and synthesis, enabling the user to obtain an improved logical understanding of the scientific and medical literature."[21]

ChatGPT clearly can provide new diagnostic and treatment possibilities that may not immediately occur to a busy clinician. But the technology behind the chatbot relies primarily on an assortment of mathematical calculations and attention mechanisms, not an innate reasoning process, at least not in the way that medical experts usually define that concept. As Rao and colleagues point out, "ChatGPT's answers are generated based on finding the next most likely 'token'—a word or phrase to complete the ongoing answer."[19] That doesn't sound like reasoning, but simply the quest to obtain statistical probability.

That's not to suggest that the technology underlying LLMs can't perform some impressive feats, especially with the help of prompt engineering. If prompts—another word for queries—given to an LLM are structured properly, or if each prompt and answer is followed by a more probing query, the results can, indeed, be impressive. Peter Lee of Microsoft, the principal investor in ChatGPT, provided ChatGPT with a detailed description of a 43-year-old-woman who presented to the ED with abdominal pain, nausea, vomiting, right quadrant pain, elevated white blood cell count, and other symptoms and signs, and asked, "What is your initial impression?" The bot provided a detailed response that suggested the physician consider not just appendicitis but ovarian torsion and ectopic pregnancy, pointing out that imaging might pin down a definitive diagnosis. Lee replied to that answer by asking if a CT scan might be inappropriate given the possibility of pregnancy, which would expose the fetus to ionizing radiation. The chatbot suggested ultrasound as a possible alternative. The two-way conversation continued, with both participants offering useful insights on the best course of action.[22]

While conversations like this have attracted the attention of many clinicians and technology developers, the question remains: Is this the kind of deep clinical reasoning that experienced healthcare experts use to make decisions? An expert clinician will take an individual medical history and perform a physical exam, and often adjust each component of the workup based on a patient's subtle physical and emotional cues. That's not something a chatbot is capable of. Clinicians are also skilled at choosing and interpreting lab tests and imaging results, which don't always conform to the recommendations outlined in the textbook cases ingested by LLMs. That interpretation involves reviewing sensitivity, specificity, area under the curve, and positive predictive value. The best clinicians are also self-aware enough to watch for a long list of cognitive biases that can influence the decision-making process. Finally, they'll take into account published clinical guidelines, scoring systems, and various other decision aids. ChatGPT, on the other hand, usually doesn't provide references to the biomedical literature or clinical guidelines for the recommendations it provides.

The debate about what's "under the hood" of LLMs will likely continue for some time. Some thought leaders point to evidence showing that these tools have logical, analytical skills that are very similar to our own. Others believe LLMs are simply good at calculating the statistics of language and can "pattern match output well enough to mimic understanding." Until this puzzle is solved, it's best to use LLMs to supplement our innate reasoning ability and clinical experience, always keeping in mind that they sometimes invent things that sound very plausible yet are inaccurate.

There are also ways to enhance the value of AI-driven chatbots and reduce their risk of generating misinformation. Chatbots like ChatGPT draw their data directly from the general internet, which contains a mountain of facts and fiction. One alternative is retrieval-augmented generation (RAG), which can control model knowledge and reduce hallucinations. The idea is simple. Clinical information from Mayo Clinic, Duke, Intermountain, and Massachusetts General Brigham is trustworthy. An LLM based on content from these sources would be far less likely to mislead users with misinformation or hallucinations, provided it has appropriate guardrails inserted by its developers.

GENERATIVE AI NEEDS GUARDRAILS

Even with tools like RAG, LLMs can still generate unreliable results, which may not matter much if you're asking it to choose the 10 best movies of all time, but can have serious consequences if you're diagnosing a life-threatening disease. The latest version of ChatGPT, version o1, which will likely be widely available by the time this book is published, is designed to address many of these problems. OpenAI, the company that makes ChatGPT, explains that the new models are designed "to spend more time thinking through problems before they respond, much like a person would. Through training, they learn to refine their thinking process, try different strategies, and recognize their mistakes."[23] Hopefully, this will reduce the risk of generating false or misleading information. OpenAI has also implemented more safety measures, putting the model through new safety training, stating: "One way we measure safety is by testing how well our model continues to follow its safety rules if a user tries to bypass them (known as 'jailbreaking').

On one of our hardest jailbreaking tests, GPT-4o scored 22 (on a scale of 0-100) while our o1-preview model scored 84."[23] In addition, OpenAI has formalized agreements with the U.S. and U.K. AI Safety Institutes.

Of course, even the most carefully developed chatbots still need safeguards to keep them from "flying off the rails." That's one of the goals of the Coalition for Health AI (CHAI), which we mentioned in Chapter 3 of this book. CHAI is a community of academic health systems, organizations, and expert AI and data science practitioners. These members have come together to harmonize standards and reporting for health AI and to educate end users on how to evaluate these technologies to drive their adoption.

CHAI recently published *The Generative AI (GenAI) CHAI Best Practices Framework Guide (BPFG)*. It aims to provide all stakeholders involved in an AI-enabled solution—healthcare providers, hospital administrators, and researchers—with best-practice guidance and a testing and evaluation framework. The *BPFG* leverages and augments the base CHAI Assurance Standard (AS) Guide—which consists of comprehensive AI assurance principles and considerations applicable at all stages of the AI life cycle—and develops operational best practices along with testing and evaluation methods and metrics.

Specific examples and use cases are described in the *BPFG* to ground best-practice concepts for real-world problems and the AI solutions implemented to solve these problems. Best practice guidance consists of actionable recommendations, protocols, or guidelines designed to ensure safe, effective, and ethical use of AI technologies in healthcare. These guidelines focus on ensuring patient safety, optimizing clinical outcomes, promoting interoperability, and upholding ethical standards in development, deployment, and monitoring of AI systems.

FINAL THOUGHTS

As we've stated throughout this book, we now have access to a wide variety of digital tools that are already having a very real impact on individual health. Smartphone apps can help detect abnormal heart rhythms like atrial fibrillation. Algorithms exist to help detect skin cancer and several other life-threatening disorders. It's also possible to detect early onset of diabetes with the help of certain digital tools, increase the detection rate for colorectal cancer, and make high-quality at-home care of cancer patients a reality. With all these tools at our disposal, the future looks bright. It's no exaggeration to say that we're entering a new era in medicine, one in which digital health will profoundly impact how you and your neighbors receive patient care and the ways in which you provide medical self-care. Welcome to the journey.

KEY TAKEAWAYS

- Generative AI has the potential to improve online conversations between clinicians and patients, help summarize a 100-page electronic health record, and perhaps even improve the diagnoses of complex diseases.

- Despite such possibilities, experts advise caution because these chatbots can generate misleading information or even invent "facts." Thus, there's a need for guardrails from regulators and the Coalition for Health AI (CHAI).

- Advances in AI are transforming healthcare and medical self-care. Smartphone apps can now help detect abnormal heart rhythms like atrial fibrillation. Algorithms can help detect skin cancer, and other computer programs are screening for diabetic eye disease and much more.

References

[1] Carle E. Ask a Techspert: What is generative AI? *Google: The Keyword.* Accessed September 25, 2024. https://blog.google/inside-google/googlers/ask-a-techspert/what-is-generative-ai/#:~:text=Large%20language%20models%20(LLMs)%20are,form%20of%20natural%2Dsounding%20language.

[2] Stanford HAI. Large language models for health 101. Accessed September 25, 2024. https://www.youtube.com/watch?v=b88FZYNJdIk.

[3] Cerrato P, Halamka J. *Redefining the Boundaries of Medicine.* Mayo Clinic Press; 2023:4.

[4] Lee A. What is a pretrained AI model? Nvidia Blog. Accessed October 2, 2024. https://blogs.nvidia.com/blog/2022/12/08/what-is-a-pretrained-ai-model/.

| 5 | Syal A. Intro to pre-trained ML APIs in Google Cloud platform. Accessed October 2, 2024. https://www.youtube.com/watch?v=1Qx2i8f-e0.

| 6 | What are transformers in artificial intelligence? Amazon Web Services. Accessed February 5, 2025. https://aws.amazon.com/what-is/transformers-in-artificial-intelligence/#:~:text=Transformers%20are%20a%20type%20of,sequence%20into%20an%20output%20sequence.

| 7 | Michael C. A layperson's guide to understanding ChatGPT's token-based pricing: The affordable way to bring conversations to life. Accessed October 3, 2024. https://mcengkuru.medium.com/a-laypersons-guide-to-understanding-chat-gpt-s-token-based-pricing-fee340d504c8#:~:text=A%20token%20is%20a%20piece,pay%20%240.002%20or%200.2%20cents.

| 8 | The AI Hacker. Illustrated guide to transformers neural network: A step by step explanation. Accessed October 3, 2024. https://www.youtube.com/watch?v=4Bdc55j80l8.

| 9 | Tai-Seale M, Baxter SL, Vaida F, Walker A, et al. AI-generated draft replies integrated into health records and physicians' electronic communication. *JAMA Netw Open.* 2024 Apr 1;7(4):e246565. doi: 10.1001/jamanetworkopen.2024.6565.

| 10 | Reisman J. I'm a doctor. ChatGPT's bedside manner is better than mine. *New York Times.* October 5, 2024. https://www.nytimes.com/2024/10/05/opinion/ai-chatgpt-medicine-doctor.html?searchResultPosition=1.

| 11 | Mouhawasse E, Haff CW, Kumar P, et al. Can AI chatbots accurately answer patient questions regarding vasectomies? *Int J Impot Res* 2024 Aug 24. https://doi.org/10.1038/s41443-024-00970-y.

| 12 | Ayers A, et al. Comparing physician and artificial intelligence chatbot responses to patient questions posted to a public social media forum. *JAMA Intern Med.* 2023. 183:589-596.

| 13 | Shmerling RH. Can AI answer medical questions better than your doctor? *Harvard Health Publishing.* March 27, 2023. Accessed October 14, 2024. https://www.health.harvard.edu/blog/can-ai-answer-medical-questions-better-than-your-doctor-202403273028.

| 14 | Gulshan V, Peng L, Coram M, et al. Development and validation of a deep learning algorithm for detection of diabetic retinopathy in retinal fundus photographs. *JAMA*. 2016 Dec 13;316(22):2402-2410. doi: 10.1001/jama.2016.17216.

| 15 | Liu X, Faes L, Kale AU, et al. A comparison of deep learning performance against health-care professionals in detecting diseases from medical imaging: A systematic review and meta-analysis. *Lancet Digit. Health*. 2019 Oct;1(6):e271-e297. doi: 10.1016/S2589-7500(19)30123-2.

| 16 | Nagendran M, Chen Y, Lovejoy CA, et al. Artificial intelligence versus clinicians: Systematic review of design, reporting standards, and claims of deep learning studies. *BMJ*. 2020 Mar 25:368:m689. doi: 10.1136/bmj.m689.

| 17 | Heaven WD. Why Meta's latest large language model survived only three days online. *MIT Technology Review*. November 18, 2022. Accessed October 14, 2024. https://www.technologyreview.com/2022/11/18/1063487/meta-large-language-model-ai-only-survived-three-days-gpt-3-science/.

| 18 | Berg HT, van Bakel B, van de Wouw L, et al. ChatGPT and generating a differential diagnosis early in an emergency department presentation. *Ann Emerg Med*. 2024 Jan;83(1):83-86. doi: 10.1016/j.annemergmed.2023.08.003.

| 19 | Rao A, Pang M, Kim J, et al. Assessing the utility of ChatGPT throughout the entire clinical workflow: Development and usability study. *J Med Internet Res*. 2023 Aug 22:25:e48659. doi: 10.2196/48659.

| 20 | Shea Y-F, Lee CMY, Ip WCT, Luk DWA, et al. Use of GPT-4 to analyze medical records of patients with extensive investigations and delayed diagnosis. *JAMA Network Open*. 2023 Aug 14;6(8):e2325000. doi: 10.1001/jamanetworkopen.2023.25000.

| 21 | Truhn D, Reis-Filho JS, Kather JN. Large language models should be used as scientific reasoning engines, not knowledge databases. *Nature Med*. 2023 Dec;29(12):2983-2984. doi: 10.1038/s41591-023-02594-z.

| 22 | Lee P, Goldberg C, Kohane I. *The AI Revolution in Medicine: GPT-4 and Beyond*. Pearson Education; 2023.

| 23 | OpenAI. Introducing OpenAI o1-preview. Accessed October 23, 2024. https://openai.com/index/introducing-openai-o1-preview/.

PAUL CERRATO, MA, is a senior research analyst and communication specialist with Mayo Clinic Platform, a technology initiative composed of solution developers, data partners, and healthcare service providers focused on finding digital solutions to many of the stubborn problems facing healthcare. In 2024, Mayo Clinic Platform tools and solutions reached over 56 million people. Cerrato also is a professor at D'Amore-McKim School of Business at Northeastern University, where he teaches data mining and machine learning.

Cerrato has served as editor of *InformationWeek Healthcare,* executive editor of *Contemporary OB/GYN,* and senior editor of *RN Magazine.* He has been published in the peer-reviewed medical literature and has written six books on digital health. Cerrato has also been named one of the most influential bloggers by the Healthcare Information and Management Systems Society, known as HIMSS. He was recently inducted into Sigma Xi, the Scientific Research Honor Society, whose past inductees include Albert Einstein, Linus Pauling, and more than 200 Nobel Prize winners.

JOHN D. HALAMKA, MD, MS, is the Dwight and Dian Diercks President of Mayo Clinic Platform. Trained in emergency medicine and medical informatics, Dr. Halamka has been involved in healthcare information strategy and policy for more than 40 years. Prior to his appointment at Mayo Clinic, he was chief information officer at Beth Israel Deaconess Medical Center and the International Healthcare Innovation Professor at Harvard Medical School.

A graduate of Stanford University, Dr. Halamka earned his medical degree at the University of California, San Francisco. He also pursued graduate work in bioengineering at the University of California, Berkeley. Dr. Halamka completed his residency in emergency medicine at Harbor-UCLA Medical Center. He continues to practice emergency medicine, while also serving as a professor of emergency medicine and the Michael D. Brennan, MD, President's Strategic Initiative Professor at Mayo Clinic College of Medicine and Science. Dr. Halamka has written 15 books and numerous articles and, in 2020, was elected to the National Academy of Medicine. He and his wife run Unity Farm Sanctuary in Sherborn, Massachusetts, dedicated to the lifetime care of ill, disabled, senior, orphaned, and surrendered farm animals.

Index

Scan to learn more about
Mayo Clinic Platform
and the future of healthcare